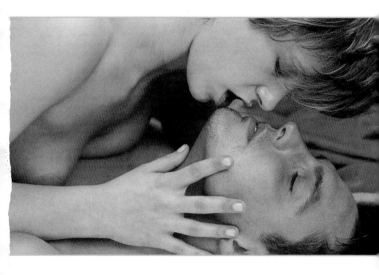

CONNOISSEUR'S
SEX
GUIDE

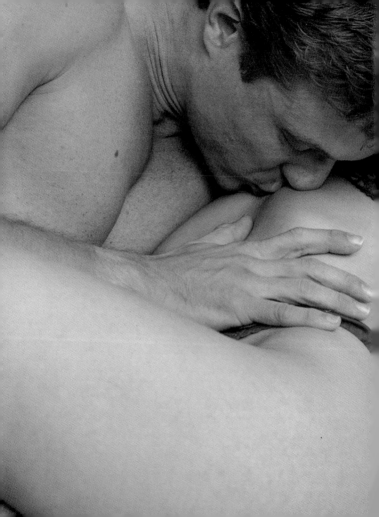

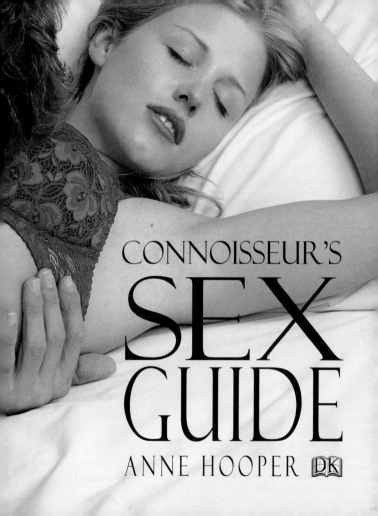

CONNOISSEUR'S SEX GUIDE

ANNE HOOPER **DK**

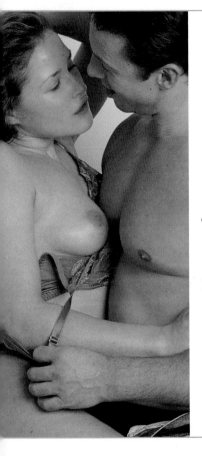

London, New York, Munich,
Melbourne, Delhi

BRAND MANAGER FOR ANNE HOOPER
Lynne Brown,
SENIOR ART EDITOR Helen Spencer,
DESIGNER Carla De Abreu,
BOOK EDITOR Jane Cooke,
DTP DESIGNER Traci Salter,
PRODUCTION Louise Bartrum

Art Director Carole Ash
Publishing Director Corinne Roberts

Published in the United States by
Dorling Kindersley Publishing, Inc., 375
Hudson Street, New York, New York 10014

2 4 8 10 9 7 5 3

Copyright © 2005 Dorling Kindersley Limited
First published as a part of *Sexopedia* in 2003
Text copyright © 2003, 2005 Anne Hooper

The rights of Anne Hooper to be identified
as Writer of this Work have been asserted
by her in accordance with the Copyright,
Designs and Patents Act, 1988.

All rights reserved. No part of this publication
may be reproduced, stored in a retrieval
system, or transmitted in any form or by any
means, electronic, mechanical, photocopying,
recording, or otherwise, without the prior
permission of the copyright holder.

A CIP catalog record for this book is available
from the Library of Congress

ISBN-13: 978-0-75661-345-7
ISBN-10: 0-75661-345-0

Colour Reproduction by Colourscan, Singapore
Printed and bound in Singapore
by Tien Wah Press

See our complete catalogue at
www.dk.com

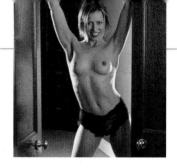

Introduction

ONE OF THE CHALLENGES loving couples
can encounter is knowing how to show their
love more freely. They long to go further
physically and their desire is part of the
intense passion they feel for one another.

Some lovers find it difficult to show
the strength of their passion because, in
order to become truly sexually intimate,
they need to feel they can be themselves
entirely and that their adored partner
totally accepts them – just as they accept
their lover in return.

Inhibition or inexperience may make
partners frightened of spoiling an already
wonderful relationship. Perhaps they
know there are daring sexual activities
to explore and would like to try them but
don't know how.

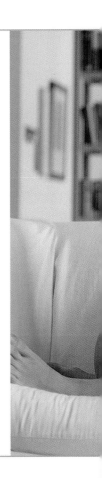

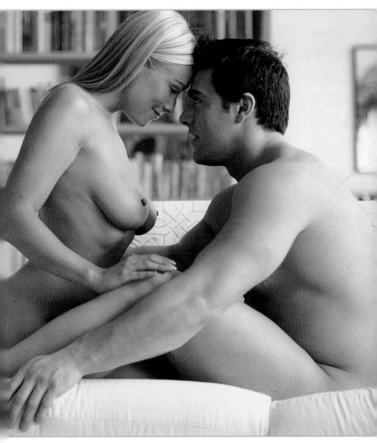

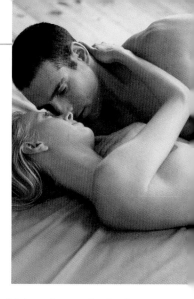

This book is for couples who want to explore one another that little bit further. It builds on well-known sex techniques and moves on to explore bold new kinds of erotic experience.

The many and varied sex positions, role plays, tricks, games, and fantasies that feature on these pages aren't just pleasure rewards. More importantly, they can be windows on a lover's mind – multiple pathways that lead to increased experiences of adoration and understanding between two loving partners.

Eastern examples of sexual practices are featured to inspire fresh approaches. Tantric sex, for example, is based on the principle that a state of mind and body ecstasy can be achieved through intercourse. For couples who are helplessly carried away with one another there are more daring techniques for

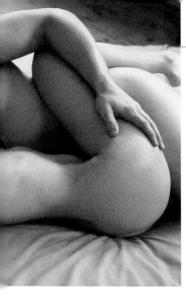

achieving multiple orgasms and for anal stimulation.

When you try a sexual activity for the first time, you move your boundaries. You express your absolute trust and adoration for a partner by becoming a "sexual explorer".

But it takes some people longer than others to get comfortable with new ideas, so always take the pressure off when a lover expresses doubt. When a love affair works really well it's because lovemaking embodies this understanding.

Dare to express your love through sex...and dare to hold back when your lover wants you to – both are part of the most intensely erotic love affairs.

Anne J. Hooper

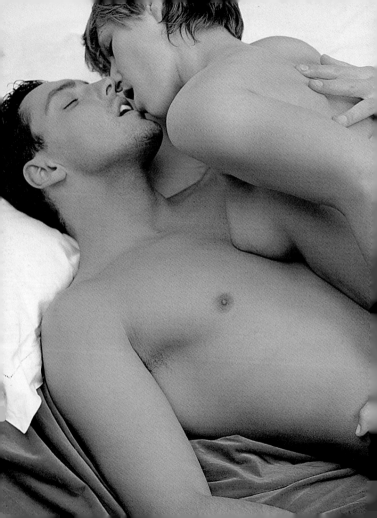

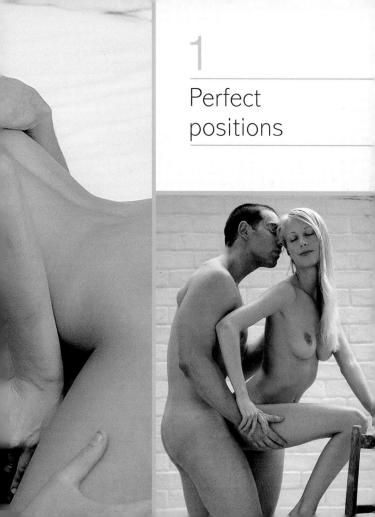

1

Perfect positions

Man-on-top positions

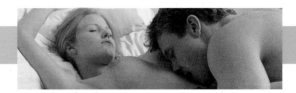

Sexual positions in which the man is on top have long been favoured by couples in the Western world. This is possibly because they are the most **comfortable** and conserving of energy; in addition, they are among the positions in which the woman is most likely to climax. They are also very **romantic**: they provide close, **face-to-face contact**, and offer you the opportunity to kiss, caress, and murmur into your lover's ear while watching his or her reaction. The missionary position is by far the most **common sex position** in European and American cultures.

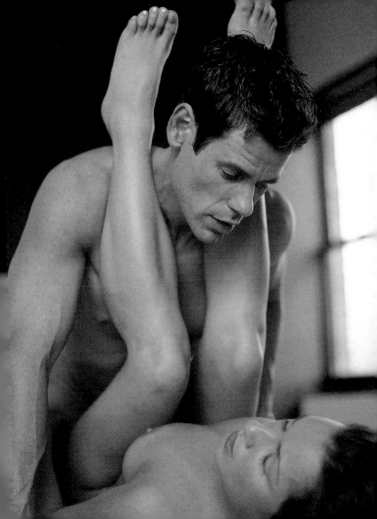

Good sex is good fun

The most important message about sexual intercourse is not to take it all too seriously. Good sex is really about having fun. So the points that follow here are not about technique – they are just general reminders that sexual intercourse is play rather than work:

1 Sexual intercourse isn't a race. There's no hurry to "complete the job", and you can take your time. Make sure that you allow plenty of time for foreplay, and make your thrusting movements as slow as you want. Most people find that they like starting off slow, but that as they get more aroused, the action spontaneously speeds up.

2 Have breaks if you want them. Some of the best sex sessions are those where you talk, laugh, and fool around, without feeling you have to "get on with it". There's no rule that specifies once you have begun thrusting you must continue to the bitter

end. Remember, your partner may get enormously stimulated by talking and laughing during sex, because that actually heightens his or her pleasure.

3 A partner usually likes to get some kind of indication that he or she is having an impact, so don't forget the importance of moaning, sighing, kissing, and saying "I love you". Sex communication doesn't just depend on your own temperament, it also depends on the kind of communication "fit" that the two of you create in the early days of the relationship, so share your feelings with your partner early on.

Varying positions

One variation on the missionary position
is for the woman to put her legs straight
out in front and closed together once
intercourse has begun. This offers an
intense method of holding the labia
bunched firmly against the penis so
that they gain maximum stimulation.

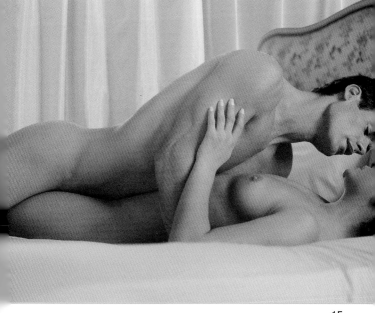

The missionary position

Legend has it that this position was so named by South Sea islanders, who spied on their local European missionaries making love. They were amused to see that the man was always on top, and found the missionaries' movements unvarying and limited. Accustomed to a more outdoor, physical life, the natives were naturally more athletic and able to sustain more energetic forms of intercourse. However, there is much to be said for this position, being both relaxing and intimate. In the basic missionary, the woman opens her legs, with her knees bent, and the man or woman guides his penis into her vagina. The beauty of the missionary is that it allows the man to support himself on both knees and

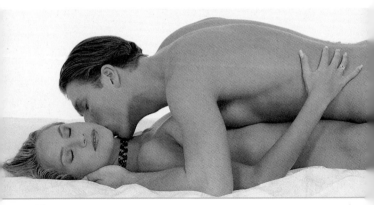

one arm, thus preventing his partner from being crushed and freeing up the second arm for amicable activity. There are many variations on the basic missionary.

Relaxed and intimate

In this variation the woman keeps her legs open but lays them out flat. This enables the couple to focus on intimacy, gentle stroking, and face-to-face contact rather than frenetic sexual activity.

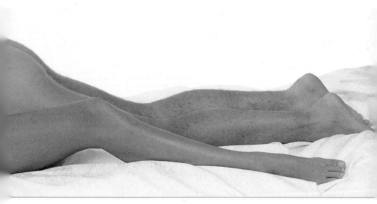

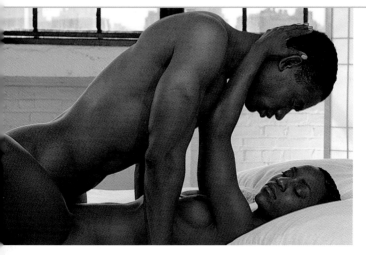

Varying the weight

Many men and women are excited by the idea of crushing or being crushed by their partner's body. There's a sensuality to the hardness and the closeness that extreme body contact provides. However, if the man on top is considerably heavier than his female partner, it may be necessary to vary the sex position to prevent her from being injured. This doesn't necessarily mean changing position entirely. He could still stay on top, but could lift himself up occasionally on his arms so that his full weight is not bearing down on his partner.

Supporting his weight

He takes the weight off her by raising himself up on his arms, while she tenderly strokes his neck and head.

Sex tip

Women – once your man has raised himself up on his arms you may miss the intimacy of body contact. To get closer to him, raise your hips up high so that your pelvis presses up against his.

Intimate wraparound

This position, where the couple lie very close and tightly against one another, shows intimate tenderness and passion.

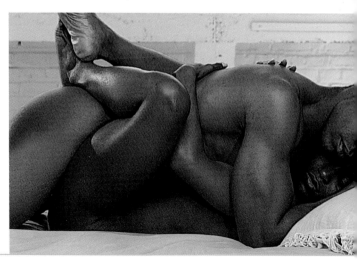

Elevating her legs

Sexual intercourse often creates some very primitive feelings in couples, particularly the desire to get as close as possible to another individual. It's very likely that this extreme need for closeness is an unconscious desire to get back into the womb again. One way of feeling particularly close is for the woman to lift her legs up high so that her partner has little to block his penetrating action. This allows him deep inside her body and offers him total sensation to the penis. Remember, she may need some additional manual stimulation.

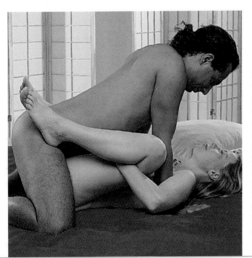

1 She eases the way
The missionary position is wonderfully changeable. You can begin with the basic position, with her feet flat on the bed or floor, and as you sensually slide together, she can slowly lift up her legs to create different sensations.

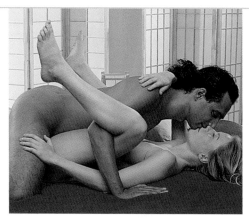

2 Supporting her legs

It can feel insecure for a woman to have her legs waving in the air, so her partner might help out by wedging his arm behind her raised knee. This allows her to rest her leg in the crook of his arm instead of straining to keep it aloft on her own.

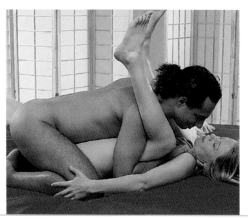

3 Maximum closeness

The man now relaxes, letting his weight down onto his elbows. This has the advantage of placing his chest pleasingly along her body, giving an intense feeling of closeness. In addition, the couple's faces are close enough together to enable passionate kissing.

Woman-on-top positions

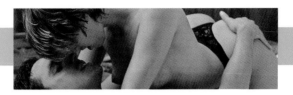

There are many advantages to woman-on-top positions. They allow the woman to be an **active participant** and to retain a **sense of control**, enabling her to set the tempo, movement, and **depth of penetration**. In addition, she can arrange the angle of thrusting so that her clitoris is in the direct line of fire and achieves **optimum pleasure**. The woman may initiate sex by sliding on top of the **erect penis** she has just coaxed into life; alternatively, the man begins on top and then the couple roll over, reversing their positions.

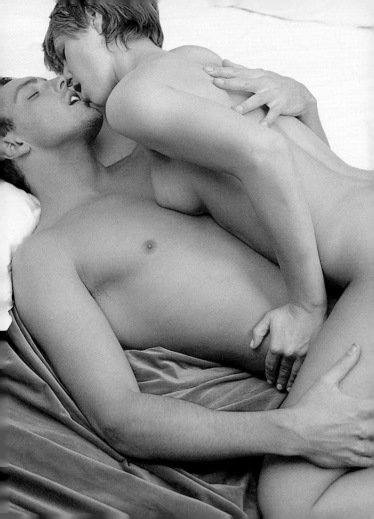

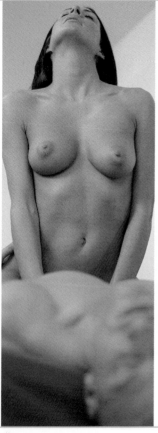

Sitting upright
Lovemaking while sitting in an upright position enables the woman to control her degree of stimulation.

Sitting astride

In Western cultures, the position in which the woman sits astride the man while facing him is probably second in popularity to the missionary position. A 1974 survey showed that nearly three-quarters of all married couples used this sexual position, at least occasionally. This figure had increased since the 1953 Kinsey Report, when only one-third of couples had said they used this position.

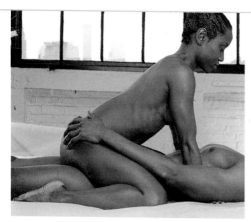

Leaning forwards

The forward angle of the woman's body means that her clitoris is able to come into contact with her partner's body. Since the woman is in charge of her own movement, this position is great for increasing her satisfaction.

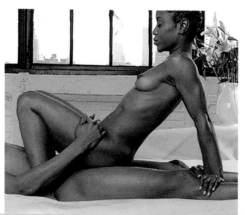

Leaning backwards

The woman can lean back, with her hands supporting the weight of her body, while continuing to move. This is a good way to slow the pace of a more thrusting sexual position.

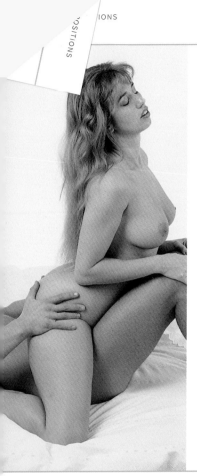

Back to front

If you only think of sexual
intercourse as a way to achieve
the ultimate goal of orgasm,
you're missing out on most of
the fun! Some of the best sex
takes place when two people are
both just enjoying each other's
bodies and experimenting with
new sensations. Couples fool
around with all kinds of unlikely
sex positions for the sheer
pleasure of it, not for the specific

Lift and support
As she rises and
falls, support her
with your raised
knees and your
hands to help aid
her movement.

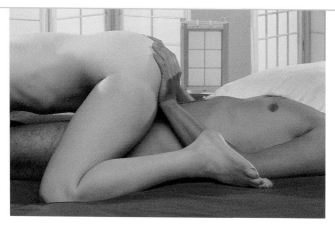

aim of achieving orgasm.
Back-to-front sex is often a
stepping stone on the way to
other more arousing sexual
positions. In the Eastern classic,
The Ananga Ranga, Kama's
Wheel is a woman-on-top
position where the woman
effectively moves full circle
around the man's penis, just for
the fun of being athletic and
experimenting with the new.

Lying on top

Be careful to avoid sudden movements
in this head-to-toe position because
the unusual angle might cause the
penis to slip and catch. But he'll love
being able to watch you move on him.

Sex tip

Increase the force of your orgasm
by putting it off for a while. The
longer you encourage arousal, the
greater the climax you will achieve.

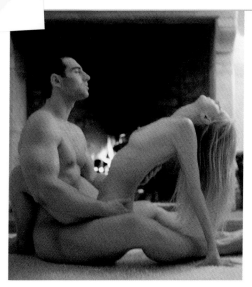

Squeezing the thighs
A gentle way to achieve pleasure is for the woman to sit astride her man, rhythmically squeezing and letting go with her thighs. This pleasures his penis while stimulating her clitoris.

Sitting positions

One of the secrets of female orgasms is that women often respond best to a steady pressure or rhythm instead of the more forceful thrust of intercourse. The bonus of woman-on-top sitting positions is that she can direct the sex – she's in charge. According to the level of sensation she's experiencing, she can speed up or slow down, move towards orgasm, or hold off from climaxing until she's ready.

Sex tip

During penetration, position the clitoris against the base of the penis. Rub softly side to side, and round and round, so that the clitoris is stimulated by the pressure.

Sitting on top

While sitting on top and facing away from your partner, you can use the strength of your thigh muscles to help you push up and down on your man's penis.

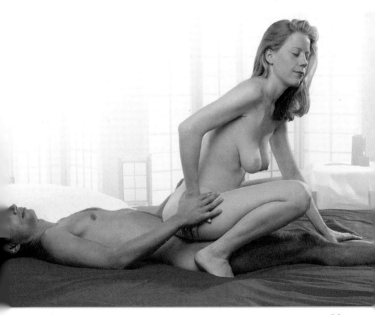

Maximizing pleasure

Caressing, stroking, and using massage can all be erotic when used on their own. They can also enhance the experience of intercourse if you can carry them out in addition to, and during, lovemaking. A good lover continues to stroke and caress his or her partner, and includes a loving touch to the genitals even during the thrust of intercourse.

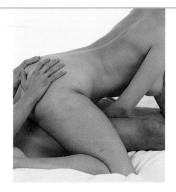

Stimulating him
To increase sensation for him during intercourse, reach down in front of you with your hand and grasp the base of his penis firmly. As you make love, grip and simultaneously move your hand.

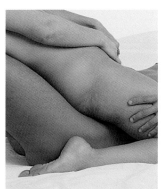

Self-stimulation
For her to achieve more sensation during penetration, she could try stroking her clitoris. Time the strokes with the thrusts of intercourse.

Points to remember

In sex, there is no contest and there is no race. The best sex is timeless and, in order to make it feel so, it's worth remembering a couple of points:

1 Try and arrange to have sex at a time of day when you're not tired. If you have more energy, there won't be so much hurry to finish – you can enjoy leisurely lovemaking.

2 Make sure your sex session is open-ended, so that you can really become absorbed in what you're doing.

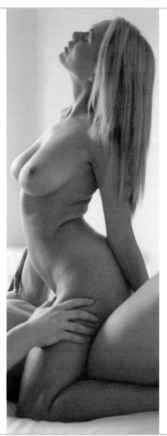

A little extra for him
The area between the anus and penis is full of nerve endings. Reach behind you, down between his legs, and cup and stroke his testicles from underneath.

Rear-entry positions

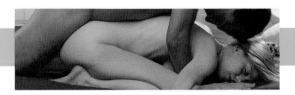

Sex from the rear feels exciting because it contains a taste of the **forbidden** and it ties neatly into **games of submission**. Both sexes find it extremely erotic – many women adore it because it makes them feel helpless; men tend to love it because the **sensation** of **thrusting** immediately below the **buttocks** is a turn-on. Some women can **climax** from sex in this position, while others manage it with some help from their partner's hands.

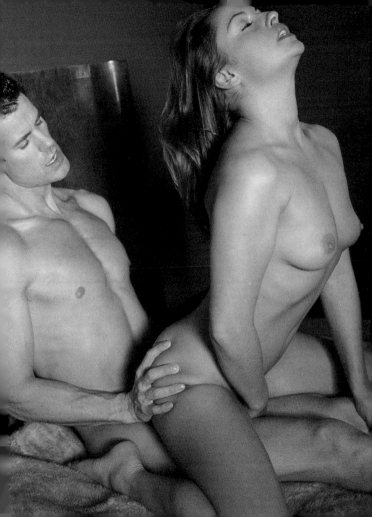

Lying down

This is an especially affectionate love position because your entire body is spread out along your partner's body, your head is next to his or hers, and you can kiss and whisper to each other during intercourse. The male pelvis rests at the rear of her buttocks and pivots from that angle, which means it is an easy and unstressful position for leisurely, rhythmic, and sensuous sex.

However, this is not a position that is likely to greatly excite your woman. By virtue of the male weight lying on top of her, she cannot really move that freely. This means that she is

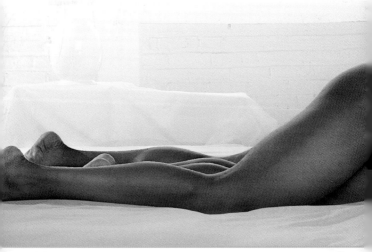

unlikely to gain any clitoral pleasure. Nor is it easy to stimulate her from underneath with your hand, since the weight of both of your bodies tends to prevent you from moving your hands easily.

Having said that, this position is great for those times when she feels like taking a more passive role, or as follow-up sex, when she has already climaxed but wants to continue enjoying the intimacy of lovemaking.

Face down

If you're a man on top, avoid resting your whole weight on your partner's body. Support some weight on your elbows.

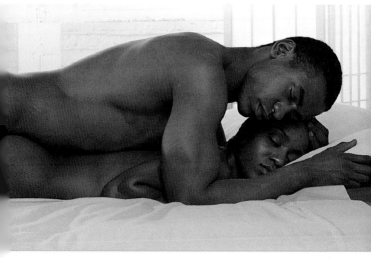

hion

uising
her ribs, slip
a cushion
underneath her
chest. This can
also help improve
the angle of
penetration.

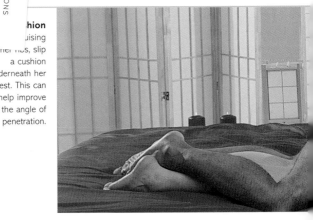

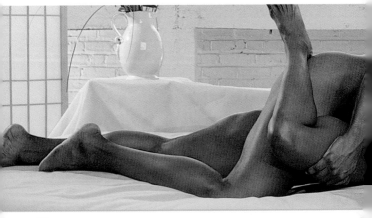

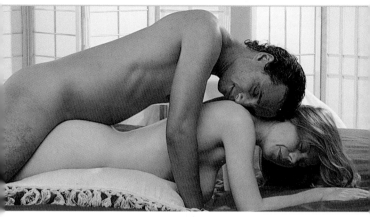

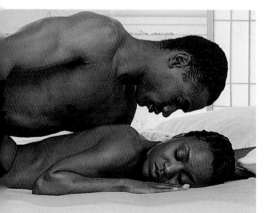

Lifting a leg

If the woman lifts her leg from the knee, it stretches her vagina slightly, opening it more widely. This increases the chances of clitoral arousal.

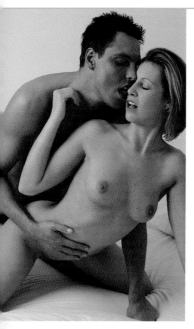

Kneeling

Probably the most comfortable of all the rear-entry positions is the one in which the woman kneels on the floor with her upper half resting on the bed and the man kneeling behind her. However, this position can prove unsatisfying for the woman. And with her thighs resting up against the side of the bed, it can be difficult for the man to reach her clitoris and stimulate her with his hands and fingers. The alternative position, doggy style on the bed, gives the man considerably more mobility and more opportunity to stimulate her genitals.

Doggy style

In this position, she can use her arms to steady herself against his thrusting, yet she can raise herself up easily for closer, more intimate contact. He has easy access to her clitoris and plenty of manoeuvrability.

Sex tip
Women – if you don't get enough stimulation from doggy-style sex, reach down and stroke yourself during sex.

Standing up

Some of the more unusual sex positions recommended in the Kama Sutra involve rear-entry sex where both parties are standing up. The Elephant is the classic pose. This is where the woman stretches down and touches the ground with her hands while her partner stands, penetrates, and thrusts from behind.

In order for this technique to work, the man must hold his partner firmly with both hands around the hips and pull and let go rhythmically, since she will be unable to make any real movements of her own. As well as being fun, this position can be used as an exercise in balance.

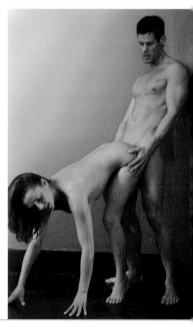

The elephant
This position can be an erotic adventure for him, but it's likely to send the blood rushing to her head, so don't pursue it for too long.

Side-by-side positions

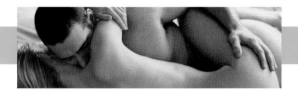

Lovemaking side by side is highly **pleasurable and relaxing**, and really comes into its own when one or both partners are physically frail, injured, or just plain tired, because it puts **less strain** on the body than other positions. It's also a **great boon** for **pregnant women** because the mattress can **support** the weight of a heavy abdomen.

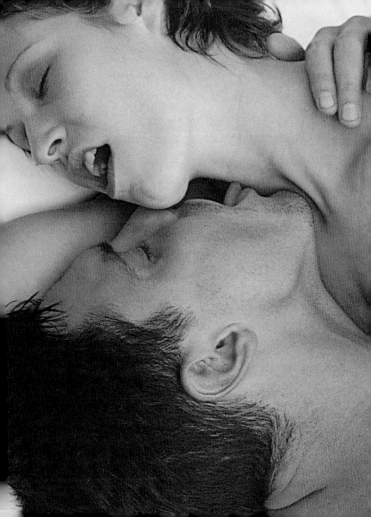

Both legs wrapped around him
One way the woman can assist her mobility is to wrap her legs around her partner's buttocks so that she can thrust against the weight of his body.

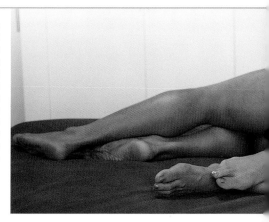

Face to face

Couples adore kissing, snuggling up, and murmuring loving words to each other. Doing this face to face is always more intimate and meaningful than back to back. It is attractively casual to just hold each other, quietly talking. Some couples doze off together in this position and wake to find themselves tightly and sexily clasped — a good starting point for making love.

As with most side-by-side positions, the face-to-face position is lazily sensual, intimate, and extremely restful, giving lovers a break if they find sex tiring. It is also recommended as a good way of prolonging intercourse and slowing down orgasm.

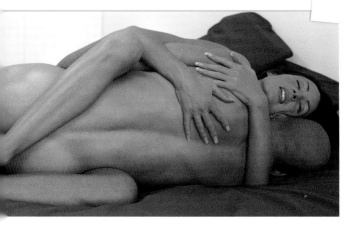

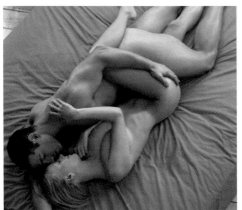

Legs intertwined

One of the sexiest sensations in bed is of stretching out and casually winding your legs around those of your partner. The legs, particularly the inner thighs, are full of sensitive nerve endings.

From behind

It is probably our primitive instincts that make us become sexual at the sight and sensation of a mate's buttocks. Among primates, the anal region gives a focal sexual signal, and humans are almost certainly no different from their monkey cousins. It's a good reason why cuddling in the spoons position brings on a regular reaction – that of becoming turned on. The great advantage of doing this while lying down is that it conserves energy.

Spoons position
When the man cuddles up closely to the woman's buttocks from behind it is usually a great turn-on for both partners and can lead easily to intercourse from the rear.

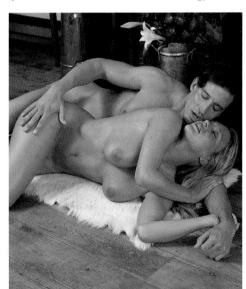

The sexual dance

At its best, sexual intercourse can resemble a wonderful series of flowing movements. There are rare but blissful occasions where physical sensation is so heightened that every action, movement, and stroke feels as though you're floating. This is the result of every nerve cell in the body being so stimulated, both by touch and by suggestion (the brain is a very sexy organ indeed), that movements can glide from one to another effortlessly, and every single action feels sensational. The real skill is to remain within that floating sensuality for as long as possible and to avoid breaking the spell with sudden or jerky movements.

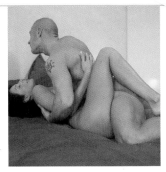

Clasping and stroking
During the best sex, any touch can bring on delicate prickles of exquisite sensuality. The stroking may be combined with moving through several sex positions, each creating more arousal.

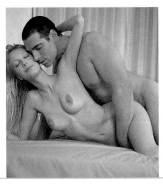

Turning and twining
The erotic dance may involve twisting around each other's bodies, an activity that stimulates nerve endings in the skin.

Kneeling positions

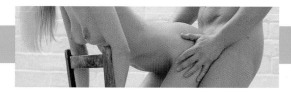

The **best** sex comes **spontaneously**, when you and your partner pick up on each other's emotions and desires and start to create a cycle of **increasing arousal**. Good sex becomes like a **wonderful dance**, with one partner following where the other leads. Try leading your partner into **experimenting** with some different **techniques**, such as these kneeling positions.

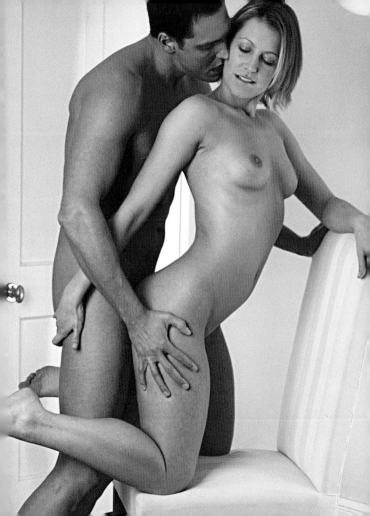

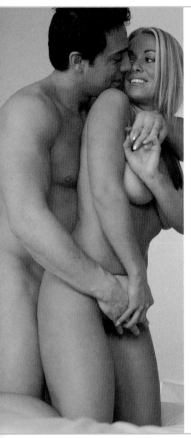

Close caresses

Any sex act that starts off by simply getting into a kneeling position is unlikely to be a great success. Embracing and kissing your partner while you're both upright feels wonderful. Then, try kneeling down together. One partner could kneel behind the other – the man could press himself against his partner's back, while caressing her with his hands.

Sex tip

To add variety to your lovemaking, start off caressing each other while you're both standing. Move into a kneeling position, and follow this with sex from the rear.

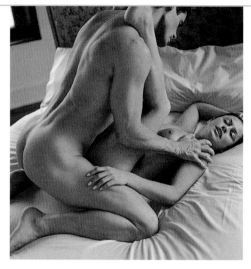

Passionate thrusting
In this position, the man is able to thrust deep inside his partner. However, the woman may find that her clitoris is not stimulated because her movement is restricted.

Deep penetration

One of the best ways to achieve deep penetration is for the woman to lie on the bed and the man to kneel up against her while she lifts her legs and places them against his shoulders. This allows him to thrust deep inside her so that he feels completely contained and she feels vulnerable and possessed. Men are especially aroused by female legs and the beauty of this position is that her legs are in full view. They can also be draped or clasped around him.

Being spontaneous

Some of the best kneeling positions are enjoyed when you are having sex in a room other than the bedroom. The sensation of being nude in the living room or kitchen can feel deliciously forbidden, and so a degree of discomfort can be forgotten in the throes of passion. In the back of the mind, there may always be the additional thought of

The novelty factor

Many people tend to follow a sexual pattern or routine with a partner – favouring positions or techniques that they have both become comfortable with. However, most of us enjoy and respond well to novelty. To spice up your love life, experiment with a few alternative positions once in a while. Try sex while kneeling in a variety of ways – it can add a new angle to your lovemaking.

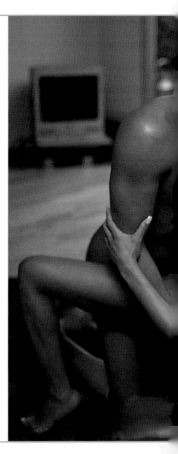

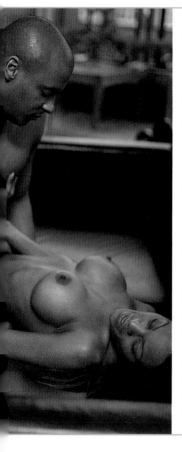

On the edge
With your partner
lying on a sofa,
kneel on the floor
next to her so that
you can get the
perfect height
and angle for
penetration.

being discovered, adding a
special "frisson" to lovemaking.

Experiment with using props
for your lovemaking, too.
A chair, for example, or the
edge of a sofa, can prove useful
props to intercourse in kneeling
positions. Sex on the edge of a
kitchen table may not be entirely
satisfactory because kitchen
tables are hard and lovers don't
respond well to discomfort, but
often it is the idea of what you
are doing and where you are
doing it that raises the eroticism
and arousal levels.

Sitting positions

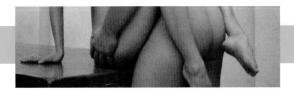

Sitting positions don't always give as much sensation as the more traditional man-on-top or woman-on-top positions, but there is something **outrageously casual** about **seated sex** that can be extremely erotic as well as great fun. You could enjoy these positions when clothed, or you could just **hint** at them when dressed to **turn your partner on**. Be aware that sitting positions can be very tiring, so don't be **surprised** if, halfway through something wonderful, your woman needs to have a change.

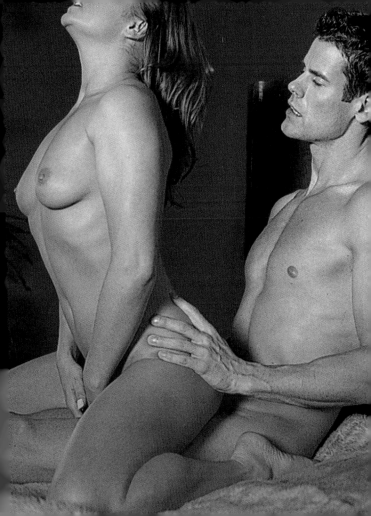

Comfort first

There are some sitting positions that are best made with a lot of back support, such as an armchair or a deeply cushioned sofa. Although it is usually the partner on top who is the more active, in some sitting positions it may be difficult to undertake certain movements without help. If she is on top she can control the angle of the thrusts (she may lean back for example), while he can move energetically and assist her movement with his hands. This has the bonus of making her feel arousingly manipulated.

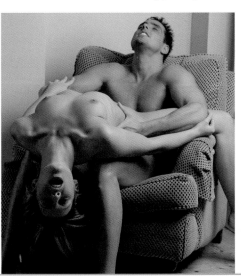

Arching back
While she is leaning back in dramatic fashion, making herself supremely open and vulnerable to his thrusting, he supports her body and helps to control the speed of motion.

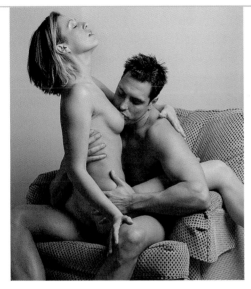

Easy access

In this position the man can reach out easily to kiss or caress his partner's breasts, buttocks, waist, and hips while helping to control the speed of penetration.

Sex tip

Sex in the sitting position is ideal for impromptu sessions when time is short. It may not cause the most fantastic sensations but its eroticism lies in its novelty value and it can be a fun preliminary.

Stimulation for her

When the woman faces away from her partner, kneeling, she can control the pace and can use her free hands to stimulate herself from the front.

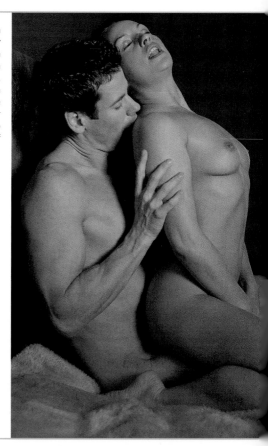

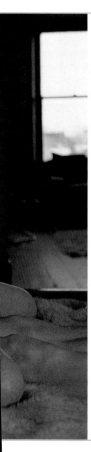

Facing away

For those couples who don't always want sex to be the height of passion with every facial flicker observed, rear-entry sex while seated offers a lazily sensual alternative. The woman sits astride the man, facing away, and takes control of the action. Her thigh muscles enable her to rise and fall and set the tempo of the thrusts. He benefits from seeing her buttocks move rhythmically, which is a powerful, primitive turn-on; indeed, the visual experience can be enough to trigger climax.

Sex tip

For rear-entry seated positions, sex therapists recommend lying back on a pile of cushions propped up against a wall. This is to provide solid support as well as comfort.

Equal partners
The face-to-face contact and proximity of this couple's bodies generate a feeling of intimacy. Both partners control the gentle rhythm and neither is dominant.

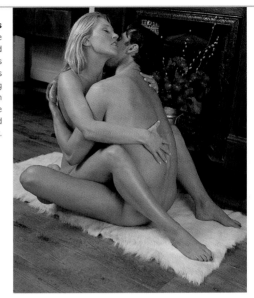

Face to face

Any face-to-face position feels supremely intimate and erotic, especially while seated, when you are squeezed up against your lover's body. A relaxed version of the face-to-face position is where the woman leans back on her arms and moves her pelvis rhythmically (this position, known as "Hector's Horse", was recorded in antique sex books).

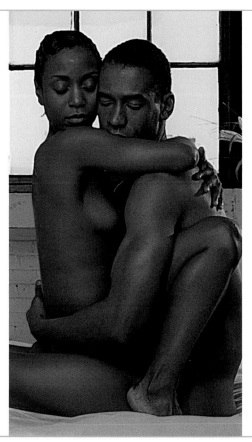

Woman in control

The woman controls the pace of lovemaking here, using her feet to provide leverage for her thrusts. The man remains fairly still and supports her body as she moves.

Upright positions

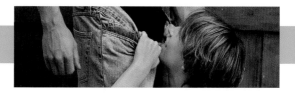

Some of the most **fantastic spontaneous sex** takes place while you and your partner are both standing upright. There is nothing quite like falling on each other in such a **rush of passion** that you don't even bother to get undressed or go to bed – you **just do it**, urgently and possessively right **on the spot**. And upright sex also comes into its own when you are suddenly **seized with desire** for each other but just happen to be in the great outdoors. There are plenty of **delicious** upright positions you could try wherever you are.

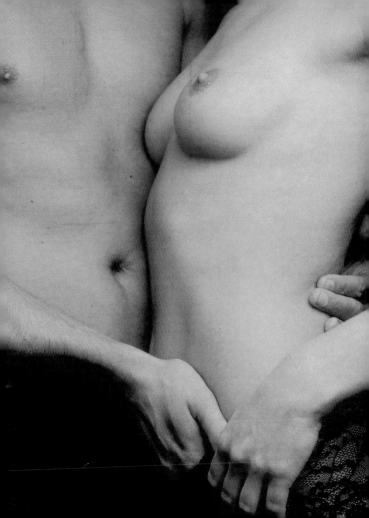

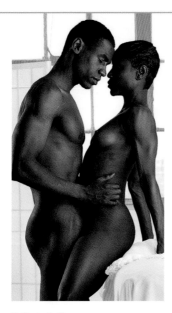

Belly to belly
Just holding each
other face to face
and belly to belly
when you are
having sex is
very sensual —
especially if you
are both naked.

Standing upright

Every slight deviation of
standing sex provides specific
sensation and special eroticism.
As he thrusts, it helps if she can
lift at least one leg upwards —
this helps to open her vagina a
little more and to envelop him
even further. If the woman
wants to take both her legs off
the ground, she might sit on a
table or otherwise be supported
by her man from underneath.

Holding up your female
partner during intercourse is a
Herculean labour of love, and
probably not one many men will
manage for very long. In the
days of the Kama Sutra, women
were sometimes pictured
clinging to their standing lovers
with their arms and legs. You
may be surprised by the strength
that passion can temporarily give
you — but don't overestimate it!

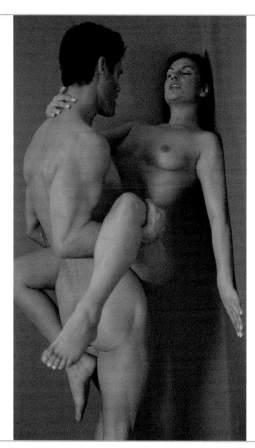

Legs entwined
It's an instinctive
urge to want
to get as close
as possible to
your man during
intercourse.
Wrapping your
crossed legs
around him
tightens the leg
muscles, draws
him closer to you,
and energizes
your pelvis.

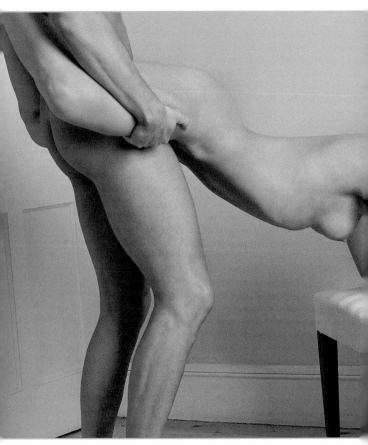

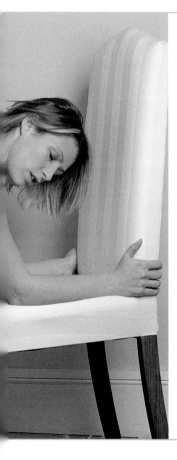

Using props

Human beings are artistic as well as inventive. By using props such as chairs or even washbasins, not only can you get yourselves into some wonderfully sensual positions, you can create imaginary erotic stories, too. Why might she be asked to raise her leg as he slips into her from the rear? What kind of a romance takes place in the bathroom over a washbasin? Let your imaginations run wild.

Sex tip

Try telling her an erotic story when you use furniture as a sexual prop. She'll turn on to the fantasy.

Wheelbarrow in the air

This position is an exciting and athletic experience, but it's not for the frail, and definitely not for women with bad backs. Don't hold it for more than a few thrusts because it might cause a back injury.

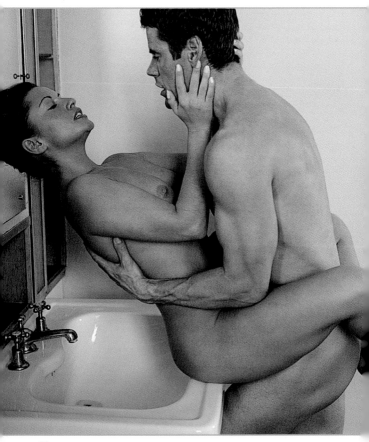

A quick wash and brush up
A washbasin is often at the ideal height for upright sex, but make sure it's secure.

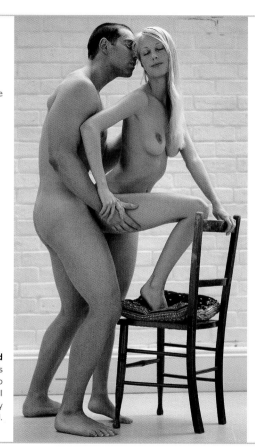

A leg lifted
If he slides his woman's leg onto a chair, she will feel erotically manipulated.

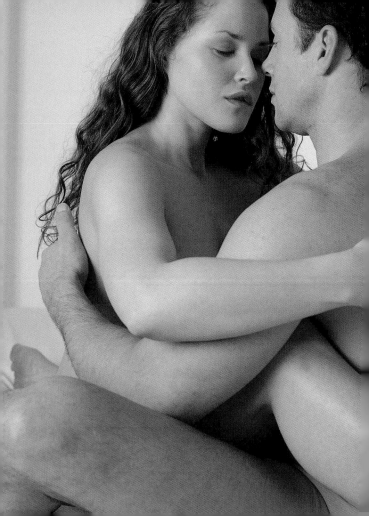

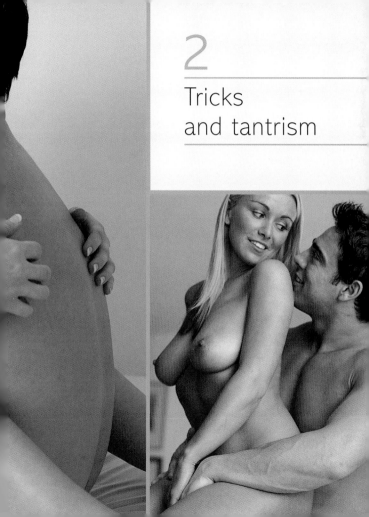

2

Tricks
and tantrism

Sex tricks

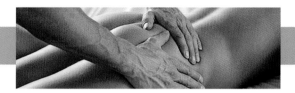

There are many things you can do to turn a mildly interesting sexual encounter into a **deeply satisfactory** one. Surprise and spontaneity in the form of unexpected sexy kisses in public, or **unusual sex positions**, can be extremely exciting. **Tender talk** is also a great aphrodisiac. Tell your partner as you **make love** how attractive you find him or her, and how much their smell or taste **turns you on**.

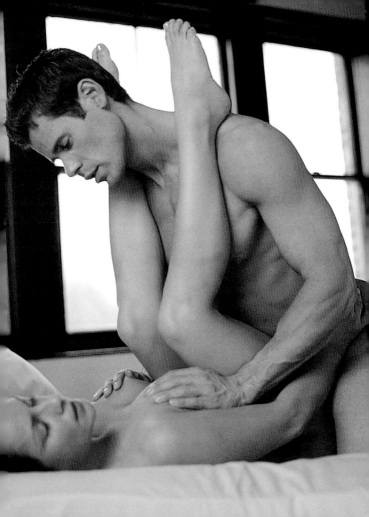

Increasing friction

A certain amount of friction is essential for sexual stimulation. Some sexual positions offer particularly close, intense contact – the grind, for example, involves the man pushing and circling inside the vagina without actually moving in and out, while the seizure technique involves the man holding back the top of his partner's pubic mound to expose the clitoris while he penetrates so that he is holding it against his penis.

Steady pressure

Deep, prolonged pressure is sometimes preferable to rhythmic thrusting, particularly for G-spot stimulation. For added sensation rub her clitoris.

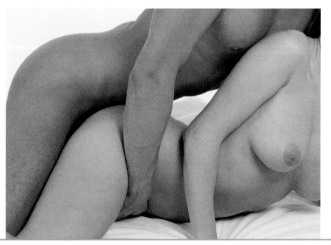

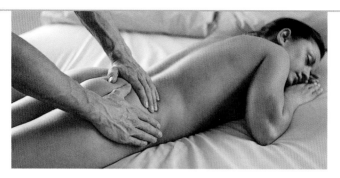

Massage during sex

One of the least exciting ways to have intercourse is to focus solely on the pounding of the penis, thereby leaving all the other erogenous zones out of the equation. The result of such single-minded thrusting is that the rest of the body ends up screaming for attention. The skin is highly sensitive, and letting your hands wander over your partner's body during intimate moments is arousing as well as loving.

Three-handed massage

Oil your partner's body, then give him or her a sensuous back massage. Let the penis penetrate the vagina while continuing with the back massage.

Sexy scent

Both men and women secrete pheromones, which are natural scent chemicals that serve to attract a mate. Pheromones travel through the air and are drawn into our systems via our sense of smell. To make the most out of your natural chemicals, don't wash as much as usual and don't wear heavy perfume.

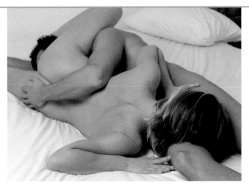

The "69" position
Simultaneous oral sex, known as the "69", is intensely intimate and requires a large degree of trust. As a result, it can be deeply satisfying to both partners.

Using your tongue

Many people aim for intercourse and often overlook the pleasures of oral intimacy. Yet skilful manipulation of the mouth and tongue on the genitals can be sensational. The "69" position describes where you snuggle up to each other head to genitals and give each other oral sex at the same time.

It is so named because of the artistic shape created by the two bodies. If you find oral sex exciting, this intimate position is a must. However, some people prefer receiving fellatio or cunnilingus separately, on the grounds that if they focus entirely on themselves rather than on their partner their sexual sensation will be more intense; equally, if they are performing oral sex on their partner separately, they can concentrate solely on giving optimum pleasure.

Sexual timekeeping

Achieving orgasm is largely a matter of timing and self-control. There are various ways that you and your partner can influence your climaxes:

• Practise peaking – this is a method of stopping then starting stimulation so that you reach mini-peaks of climax but go no further. Men and women can have many peaks in this manner before finally letting go for the big one.

• If you are aiming for simultaneous orgasm, give her plenty of foreplay and learn to let go only when you recognize what the beginning of her orgasm looks like. You may need to practise orgasm control (see pp.228–234). If you don't manage to achieve this, don't worry: most people prefer to concentrate on their orgasms separately.

• If you want to find out whether your woman is the multi-orgasmic sort, don't give up on the stimulation when she has first climaxed. Women find it very hard to regain sexual sensation if stimulation stops. Assess her physical reaction: if she is reluctant to be touched, you can guess she won't orgasm again. If she groans with pleasure and is seriously responsive, keep on with the good work. Some men can also experience multiple orgasms (see p.222–223).

Tantric sex

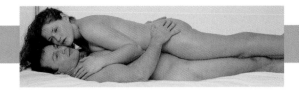

This spiritual approach to sex aims to **enrich** the **mind** and **soul** as well as provide extreme sensual pleasure. Although **tantric touch** may feel the same as other forms of touch, there is a **different emphasis** on how it is given and received. A priority of tantric sex is to **prolong sexual arousal**. It takes the form of **extensive stroking sessions** followed by very slow intercourse.

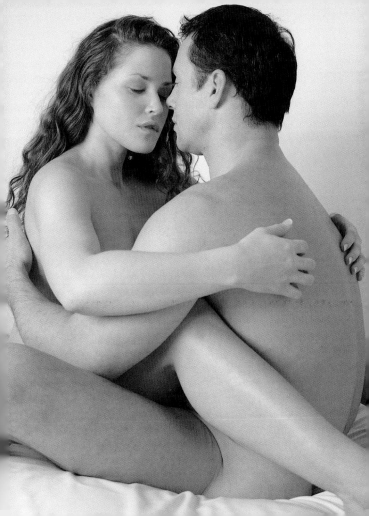

Tantric stroking

Tantric stroking, a necessary preliminary to tantric intercourse, is very similar to Masters and Johnson's sensate focus therapy. Both approaches emphasize the "touch for pleasure's sake" principle, stressing the importance of giving and receiving pleasure in a particular way. There are two sensations to be appreciated when carrying out the exercise below. The first is your own – what you feel when you touch your partner. The second is to imagine what your partner feels when touched by you. Try not to speak throughout the following series of five exercises on this page and the next.

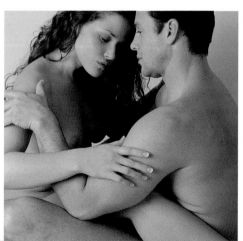

1 Lightly stroke each other, first with a circling action and then up and down. Avoid the breasts and the genitals. Stroke slowly for about 15 minutes, take a break, then repeat the stroking for another 15 minutes. Later in the evening, repeat the stroking for 30 minutes.

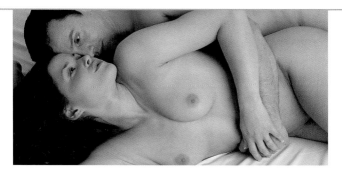

2 Lie quietly together closely in the spoons position, but without stimulating each other (if this is too tempting, lie facing each other with foreheads together but bodies not quite touching).

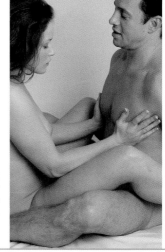

3 The next day, move on to stroking each other's chest. Make light, circular movements on the chest or breast, first with hands moving towards each other, then with the action of the hands reversed.

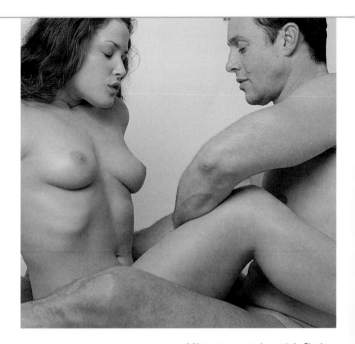

4 Next, move on to the genitals. Slowly draw your hands or fingers up from underneath each other's genitals, using very light strokes and working along the length of the penis or up the height of the vulva. Also include the testicles, perineum, vagina, labia, and clitoris.

5 After an hour of genital stroking, take a five-minute break. Then lie motionless, with the woman on top and the man's penis inside her vagina, until his erection subsides.

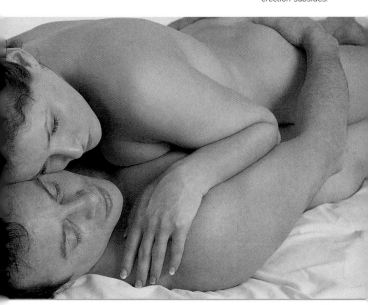

Tantric intercourse

Only once you've completed the tantric strokes do you move on to intercourse – the key is to take your time (orgasm should be put off for at least 20 minutes to half an hour). The penis should penetrate the vagina by only a few centimetres or so, stay there for a full minute, then withdraw and rest in the clitoral hood for a further minute before sliding back in. Continue with the penetration followed by a full minute's rest in between, but for the next few strokes let the penis rest outside the vulva, then on subsequent strokes just inside it. Try to imagine all the sensation your partner is experiencing as your own. Let the boundaries between you dissolve in this manner. There are various positions that

prolong intercourse or increase the pleasure of orgasm. Side-by-side positions tend to prolong intercourse (see pp.40–45), and the missionary position is also useful because the man can control an impending orgasm by pulling his testicles downward. Rear-entry positions (see pp.32–39) can be excellent for enhancing orgasm. The man can easily reach the woman's clitoris to stimulate her, and when she climaxes, his proximity to her anal muscles means that his penis will be affected by the strength of her contractions.

Three-day event

This Tantric three-day event is suitable for trying out over a long, leisurely weekend:

1 Spend the first day walking in the country, slowing down and (hopefully) feeling more peaceful. Use the lazy time spent together to renew feelings of intimacy. On the first evening, carry out the tantric strokes shown on the preceding pages, but only go as far as step 2.

2 The next morning, repeat the tantric strokes up to step 2, then stop again. In the afternoon, take another slow walk. In the evening, go back to the tantric strokes, only this time include steps 3, 4, and 5. Sleep on these strokes and refrain from having sexual intercourse.

3 The following day, repeat stages 1 to 4, and this time go on, after at least an hour of stroking and stimulation,

to have intercourse. Don't instantly go for orgasm but prolong the intercourse (see opposite). Finally, when you feel the time is right, allow yourselves to climax.
(NB: You may choose to prolong intercourse by breaking for lunch or having a sleep then returning to intercourse later in the day.)

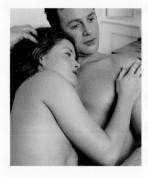

Tao of sex

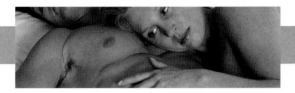

Thousands of years ago, **Tao philosophers** argued that the human body had its own **energy flow** that could be both used up and recharged, a belief that is still held by many today. They believed that by applying **stimulation to specific meridian points**, as is the case in acupuncture or reflexology, it would benefit the health of "related" organs elsewhere in the body and **restore the balance** of energy.

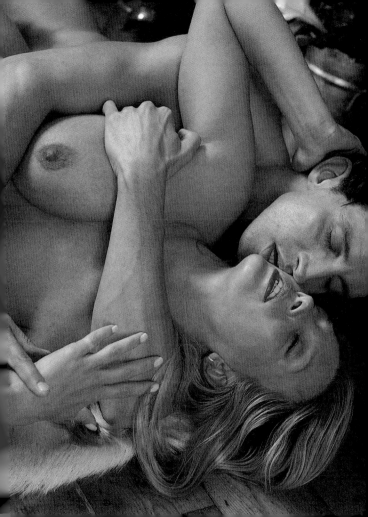

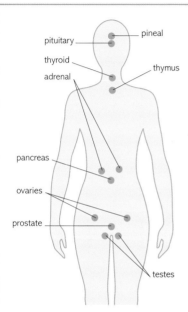

pineal

pituitary

thyroid

adrenal

thymus

pancreas

ovaries

prostate

testes

Sexy glands

In Tao philosophy, the penis and vagina are considered to possess meridian points which, if massaged correctly, will have a re-energizing effect on the glands relating to sexual function (see above).

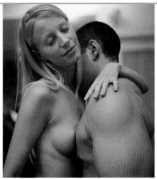

Sex for health

Tao sexual positions aim to massage the penis and vagina evenly – this is something that typical sexual intercourse does not always achieve, because of the uneven shape of the vagina and penis. The Tao genital massage, known as the Sets of Nine exercise (opposite), is made up of ninety strokes. Its purpose is to massage the genital meridian points so that all related organs in the body will benefit.

The sets of nine

In this exercise, the man penetrates his partner in a series of strokes as follows:

1 He thrusts just the tip of his penis into the vagina before withdrawing. He does this shallow stroke nine times, before thrusting the entire penis into the vagina once.

2 He then carries out eight shallow strokes (with the tip of the penis only) and two deep strokes (with the entire penis).

3 Next, he makes seven shallow strokes and three deep ones.

4 Then, he performs six shallow strokes and four deep ones.

5 He follows this with five shallow strokes and five deep ones.

6 He then performs four shallow strokes and six deep ones.

7 This is followed by three shallow strokes and seven deep ones.

8 Then, two shallow strokes and eight deep ones.

9 Finally, he makes one shallow stroke and nine deep ones.

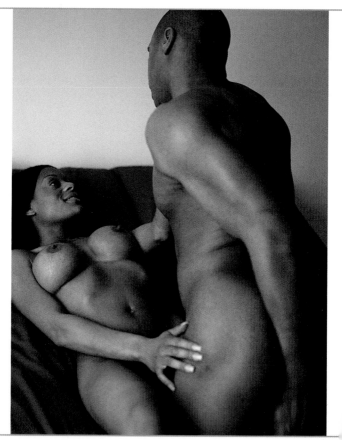

Injaculation

According to Tao theory, ejaculation can be reversed and semen re-absorbed into the man's body. Injaculation is carried out by pressing the Jen-Mo point – this is an acupressure point on the perineum, which is the area halfway between the anus and the scrotum – at the moment before ejaculation. The man will continue to feel aroused. In fact, sensation will be accentuated because the orgasm will happen very slowly – it may even continue for up to five minutes. The man will also retain his erection, or regain it quickly, and so he is able to continue intercourse for longer.

According to Tao principles, his energy will be preserved because his semen has not been expelled. Do not try injaculation if you have a prostate infection.

How to injaculate

Just as you are about to ejaculate, press your perineum so that semen is not allowed to travel through the urethra. If you apply pressure too close to the anus, it won't work. If you press too close to the scrotum, the semen will be forced into the bladder.

> ### Sex tip
>
> Try resting during intercourse without losing your erection. This is good training for lasting longer.

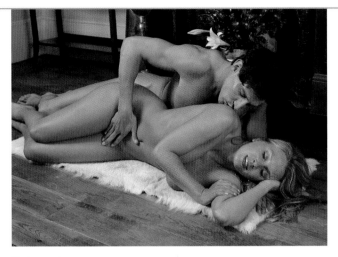

Enhancing orgasm

Tao sexology describes the female orgasm as a series of rising steps, followed by a declining step. Sensuality is built on and increased with each rising step, and these steps are known as the nine levels of orgasm. According to Tao belief, many men do not realize that there are so many stages of female orgasm. During sex, they tend to stop stimulating their partner at around Level Four (see opposite), and so the woman's climax is often curtailed. It is only through continuing stimulation that Level Nine can be reached.

Nine levels of orgasm

Each of the nine levels of orgasm energize particular parts of the woman's body. As each organ is affected, watch for the signs that show you how your partner's sensation is increasing, so that you know how to take her on through the nine levels of orgasm:

1 Lungs – The woman sighs deeply, breathes heavily, and begins to salivate.

2 Heart – While she's kissing her man, she extends her tongue out to him.

3 Spleen, pancreas, and stomach – As her muscles become activated, she grasps him tightly.

4 Kidneys and bladder – She starts to experience vaginal spasms and her secretions start flowing.

5 Bones – Her joints begin to loosen and she may even start to bite her partner.

6 Liver and nerves – She writhes and tries to wrap her arms and legs about her man.

7 Blood – Her blood is "boiling" and she tries to touch her partner all over.

8 Muscles – Her muscles completely relax. She may bite even more, and grasp her man's nipples.

9 Entire body – She collapses in a "little death", and is emotionally and sensually "opened up".

Anal sex

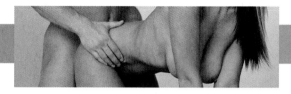

Many heterosexuals as well as homosexuals find anal sex completely natural and **spontaneously sensual** – the anal area is **rich in nerve endings**. However, there are many people who dislike the idea, considering it unhygienic, or who find it painful. It is vital to ensure that you are both **scrupulously clean**, and never go on to vaginal sex without careful washing first. A **good lubricant** is also **essential**.

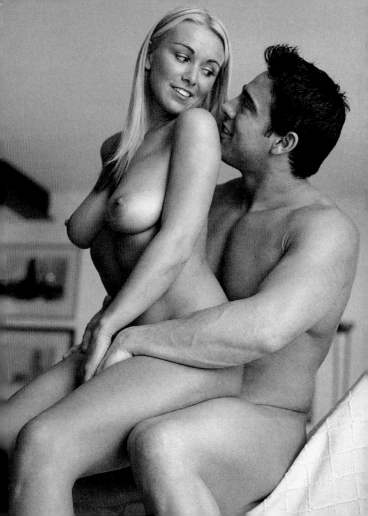

Finger massage

Moisten your fingers and your partner's anus with a suitable lubricant, such as one of the new colourful lubes (see p.141). Short, neat fingernails are essential. Massage around the outside of the anus first. As your partner becomes more relaxed, insert the tip of your finger 2–3cm (¾–1¼in) into the anus and continue to move your finger around in circles, but on the inside. Gradually make your movements firmer and use your fingertip to stretch the entrance to the anus.

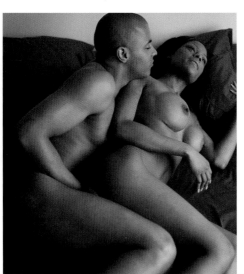

Gentle exploration
When exploring the anal area it is vital to probe gently and build up to things gradually. Check to make sure that your partner is happy for you to proceed to the next stage.

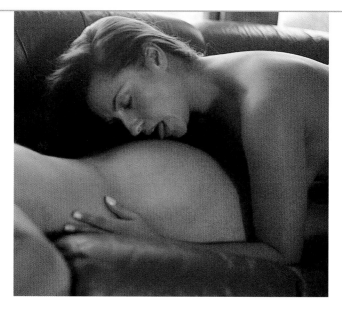

Hot spots

Think of the anus as a clock, with the 12 o'clock position closest to the vagina or testicles. The most erogenous points are usually at 10 or 2 o'clock.

Tongue bathing
The buttocks are an erogenous zone. Using your tongue to lick and probe provides a sensuous build-up to anal sex.

Taking it further

Some people prefer things to go beyond fingering around the anal passage. Many men enjoy their partner stimulating the prostate gland, which lies at the back of the anus' upper wall (see p.209); some women are profoundly turned on by a combination of fingering the anus and clitoral stimulation. Anal sex toys are very effective (see p.142–143).

If you want anal intercourse, it is vital that you are relaxed. The key to anal sex without pain is to begin by stretching the anus slowly as described on the facing page, and to use plenty of lubricant. Take penetration very gently and by degrees only. For added protection, use an extra-strong condom designed specifically for anal sex.

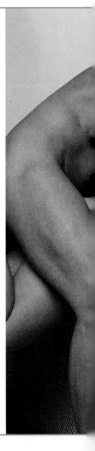

Sex tip

To make anal intercourse more comfortable, the man should pause as he penetrates so the woman can consciously relax her back passage.

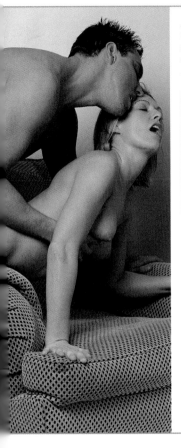

Anal intercourse

Many people, both men and women, find anal intercourse extremely exciting. Make sure the anal passage is well lubricated and sufficiently stretched before entry.

Facing objections

As with any kind of sex, never force anyone to have anal sex if they don't want to. If your partner objects to anal massage or anal penetration, you may just have to accept that it really doesn't appeal to them and explore something else instead. Sometimes a partner will feel uncomfortable with the idea but will agree to give it a try. If this is the case, take it extremely slowly and guarantee that you will stop as soon as your lover asks you to. It often helps to go back a stage so that you can discuss their anxiety and offer reassurance. To build up trust, your partner must be confident that you will stop straight away.

LEGAL WARNING: Anal sex is not legal between consenting adults in some countries and states.

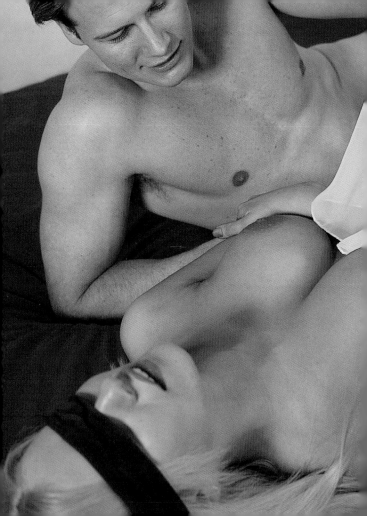

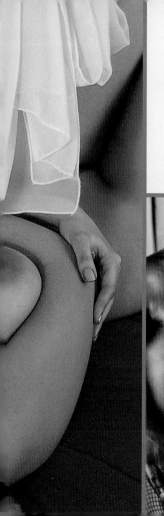

3

Roleplay
and fantasy

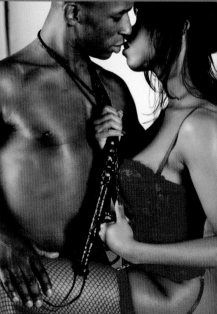

Beyond the bedroom

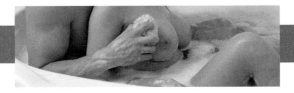

The bedroom is not the only room in the house that is **good** for **lovemaking**. Virtually any room can be an **erotic venue** as long as you are assured of privacy. The mantra to remember here is: **Go for it**. Life is too short to **make love** only in bed.

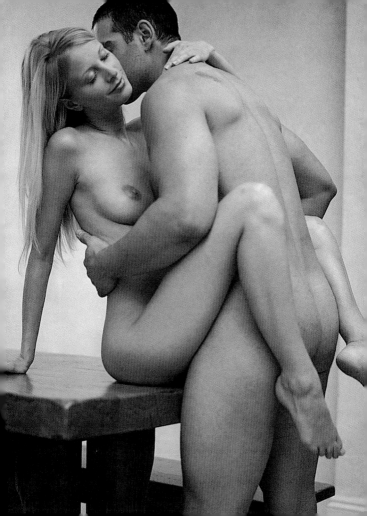

Bathroom fun

After the bedroom, the bathroom is probably the favourite room for lovemaking. Foreplay in the bath is fun and, even if your bath isn't big enough to have sex in, you can make love sitting on the edge of the tub or on the bathroom floor. Bathing before sex makes you feel clean and confident; bathing after sex enhances relaxation and intimacy.

If you are feeling tired and sluggish and you want to energize yourself before sex, spend 15 minutes soaking in a hot bath and then stand up and take a quick cold shower. Your pores will close rapidly and leave you feeling invigorated and alert. On the other hand, if you are totally stressed out, a warm bath can relax you enough to bring on lazy feelings of sensuality. Prepare the bathroom in advance with candles, a hot bath, and some fluffy towels. Now lead your partner into the steam and both get undressed. Ask him or her to step into the bath, lie back, and relax. Explain that you are going to start by washing his or her hair. Make every action as relaxing and sensual as possible.

Carry out a luxurious head massage, applying deep, circular pressure with your fingertips at the temples, the hairline, and all over the scalp. Take a comb and sensually comb his or her hair, arousing the millions of tiny nerve-endings that lie beneath the skin.

When you're bathing with your partner, try out the pelvic shampoo: wash each other's genital areas. Then swirl your fingers lightly in and out of each other's innermost crevices.

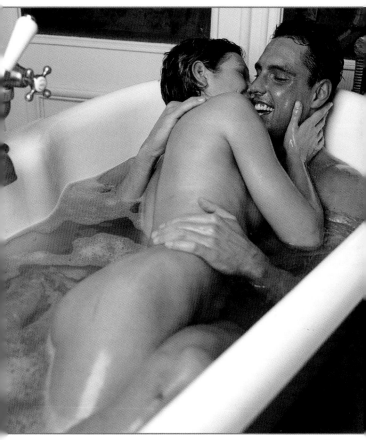

Shower games

The shower is a natural sex toy: it combines heat, pressure, moisture, and friction all in one device. There are plenty of sensual experiences you and your partner can experiment with and enjoy:

1 Play around in the shower and use the water jets on an alternate pleasure/punishment basis. Pleasure is warm water directed at the genitals; punishment is a blast of cold water on the back.

2 See if you can masturbate your woman to orgasm using only the jets of water from the showerhead.

3 Use the flow of water from the shower hose to massage different parts of the body, such as the perineum, the genitals, the toes, the lips, the soles of the feet, and the backs of the knees.

4 Cover each other in liquid soap and give each other a sensual massage.

5 Surprise your partner with some exciting oral sex in the shower.

6 If you want to try shower sex, the best position is one in which the woman bends over and is penetrated from behind.

Shower thrills

According to the Hite Report of 1974, having a shower massage is some women's favourite way of reaching orgasm. Combined with a bath, you can lie back and relax while using the shower jets to massage your erogenous zones.

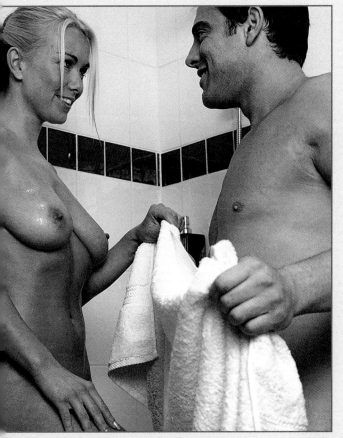

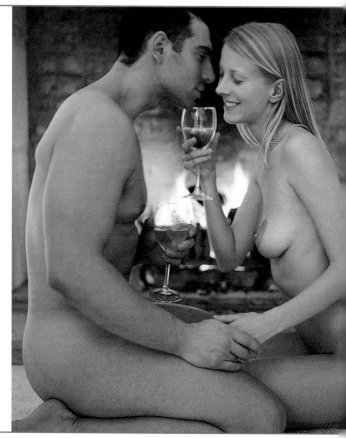

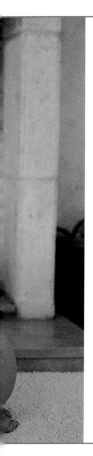

Spending an evening in front of a fire with your partner can be a sensual experience. The warmth of the fire will keep you relaxed and mellow, and the location will add a sense of adventure to lovemaking.

The living room

Any large armchair or deep-sprung sofa is an inviting spot for lovemaking, but the most erotic spot in the living room tends to be a thick rug on the floor. Preferably, this is stretched out in front of a roaring log fire!

Couples might seize the opportunity to carry out a sensual massage here, surrounded by soft music and candlelight. Single women have been known to make a night of it by locking themselves firmly in, drawing the curtains, putting some atmospheric music on, and going for a slippery self-massage in front of the fire. Single men might invest in a sexy video and go for a personal, individual, and indulgent sex party.

The kitchen

Kitchen tables are hard but for sheer change, they make an interesting venue for love. The kitchen is probably most suited for instant passion when sexual desire takes you by surprise and you can't wait a moment longer to have each other. But a word of warning – make sure you remove all sharp knives from the vicinity first!

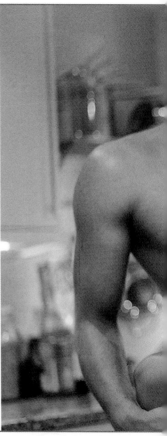

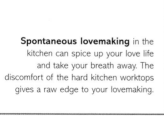

Spontaneous lovemaking in the kitchen can spice up your love life and take your breath away. The discomfort of the hard kitchen worktops gives a raw edge to your lovemaking.

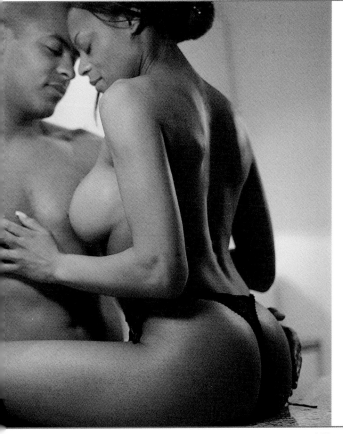

Sex outside the home

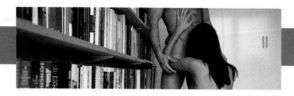

One of the great **killers of good sex** is boredom. However much you adore your partner, if you have made love in the same way, in the same bed, in the same room for years things just aren't as **erotic** as they used to be. Change only one item in that fixed pattern, such as where you **make love**, and sex takes on a new lease of life. The secret is to keep an open mind and **be unafraid** to make some slightly **different moves**.

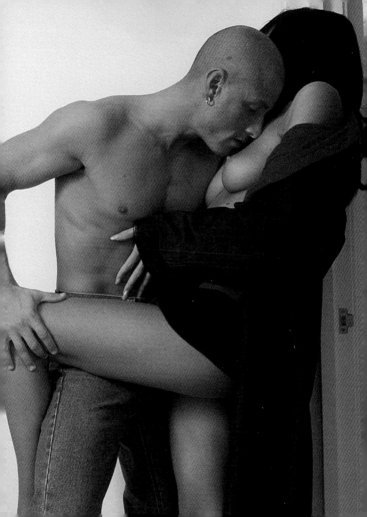

Love in the great outdoors

It's a beautiful summer's day and the two of you go for a stroll across the meadows. The sun beats down and warms your flesh and you are aware of a lazy prickling of sexual desire.

Provided you are certain that no one else can possibly see you, what could be more natural than lying down in the long grass and making love? You can hear insects humming and birds singing as you lie enclosed in this soft, green world. It's a very romantic and different experience.

Just one warning: there are laws about committing public nuisance, so it is vital to make love where you definitely cannot be observed or you might find yourself in trouble with the authorities.

Going to a hotel

Moving to a discreet hotel for an afternoon or evening can allow all kinds of unspoken fantasies to spring into reality. One woman I know presented herself at her lover's hotel room wearing nothing but her fur coat. She was faint with apprehension and when he understood what she wasn't wearing he was overwhelmed.

Another couple booked a room with a four-poster bed and spent a happy night playing Elizabethan "torture" games. The bed posts were wonderful for silken ropes, while sexy blindfolds went with the bigger picture. If your idea of luxurious sex would be to wallow in food and drink, the advantage of a good hotel is that room service will deliver goodies to your door.

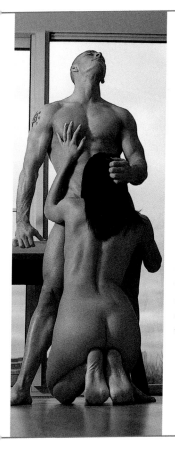

Sex in the office

Of course we shouldn't do it. The risk of a colleague finding out, even if you have closed and locked the door of the office, is high. And if this does happen, you're in trouble. Yet many people brave the possible complications for incredible experiences. One couple I know locked the office door in the lunch hour, hung out a "do not disturb" sign, and rolled around on a deep-pile rug. Another couple, who worked in an estate agency, refrained from tearing each other's clothes off in the office and instead borrowed a colleague's apartment around the corner for steamy sex.

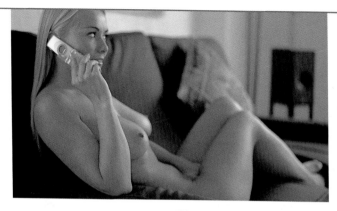

The risk factor

The risk – whether real or imaginary – of being discovered having sex can actually heighten the experience by raising adrenaline and giving an added natural chemical zap to the proceedings. However, some people get so anxious that the reaction will be a negative rather than an arousing one.

Phone sex

Anyone can dial into a sex chat line and be talked through self-stimulation. There's nothing very special about this. Nor is there anything very personal. But when you are talking erotica down the line with someone you know and like and who really turns you on that is quite different.

Before you embark on phone sex, get the circumstances absolutely right. Make sure you are unlikely to be disturbed and make the setting pleasant. Warmth, candlelight, and perfume are all delicious ingredients. Sit or lie somewhere comfortable and private, and make sure that anything you might need is within reach — you don't want to have to interrupt the proceedings.

Good phone sex

If you are missing your partner let them know it. If there are things you wish they were doing to you, voice this. Be truthful. Tell it like you are really feeling it and don't fake anything. Here are a few tips for great phone sex:

1 If there are things you know they would like done to them, let them know how you would carry out these actions if you happened to be on the spot.

2 Describe your self-stimulation as eloquently as possible. Talk your partner through what you are doing and what you imagine he or she is up to. If you use a vibrator, do so letting your man know that in your imagination he is holding this sex toy. If you are a man applying lubricant to ease the progress of self-stimulation, let your partner know that in your head this feels as if she were applying this from the very act of intercourse…your hand is her vagina, your oils are her very own sweet-smelling juices.

Exploring fantasy

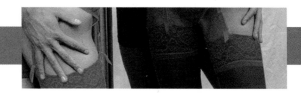

Many people love **playing games** in the bedroom, and **sharing a fantasy** is the best sort of spontaneous sex game. There are lots of ways to act out the **blue movies** of your imagination: you can wear costumes or masks, you can **use props**, you can decorate your bedroom in erotic style, or you can rely on imagination, **roleplay**, and **story-telling**.

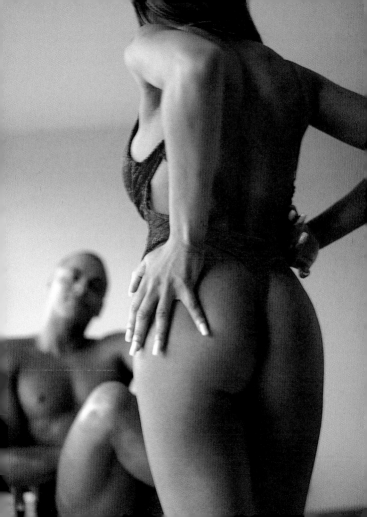

Fantasy games

Some people find it easier to liberate their imaginations and vocalize their fantasies by playing games. Somehow it helps them to become be free from their usual inhibitions. Agree any ground rules with your partner first, and then start letting your imaginations go wild!

1 On separate slips of paper, write down different fantasy roles or characters, such as a doctor or a nurse. You can also use names of famous people. Mix them up and get your partner to pull one out of a hat. Now you must both interact as if he or she is that character.

2 Choose a favourite sex scene from a film. Act it out with your partner in the same surroundings – try and use the same props, too.

3 Pick a fantasy theme and create it in your own home. For example, turn your bedroom into a palace bedroom, an Arabian tent, or a den of sex toys. If you want to transform a room quickly, the bathroom is ideal: turn the light off and just add candles, perfumed oil, bouquets of flowers, and clouds of steam.

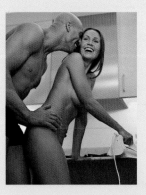

Exploring taboos

The idea of a fantasy taboo is a contradiction in terms. The whole point of a fantasy is that it is something your brain produces, virtually in spite of yourself. And yet people speak of "forbidden thoughts". We may dream of passion with someone of the same sex, or with a famous movie star. We may even dream of sex with someone "forbidden" such as a relative or a best friend's partner. Our dreams do not necessarily mean we want to make the fantasy a reality.

The notion that you can police your imagination is an old-fashioned one – you can't. But many people might take reassurance from the fact that their "unacceptable" thoughts are simply methods of exploring possibilities. They are not signs of deviance, and they would only be that if we actually went out and did the things we might have mentally pictured. And most of us don't. We experience fantasies of all sorts as a way of safely exploring something that we wouldn't actually dream of doing.

If you have a fantasy that you are nervous about, here is a game to help you: Choose one "strand" or aspect of your fantasy and explain it to your partner. The strand you choose should capture the most erotic aspect of your fantasy. For example, if you fantasize about being forced to have sex by a stranger, tell your partner that you want him to make love to you when you are least expecting it and that he must continue his seduction even if you protest.

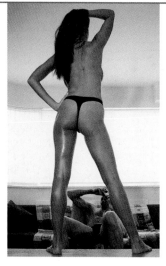

Acting out a fantasy

The beauty of sexual intimacy, especially in its early stages, is that you feel you can re-visit activities that you last considered during childhood, such as playing out imaginary roles. Many adults want to act out imaginary scenarios with their partner. Acting out fantasies is one of the teasing activities that makes a tantalized partner desperate to get as close to you as humanly possible. Since much of the essence of erotic imagination lies in the unexpected or in novelty, it is often a good idea to choose a new venue as a backdrop for your fantasy. Choose somewhere unfamiliar – a hotel, for example, or a friend's apartment.

Another benefit of sexual games is that you can stop at any stage you want. If you feel uneasy, all you have to do is call a halt. If you fear that your partner may not take your requests to stop seriously, establish a code word before you begin. And if you fear that your partner might not honour this code word, you should respectfully decline to play.

Top four fantasy roles

There are a number of fantasy scenarios that you and your partner can play out together. Take it in turns to be the submissive or dominant characters:

1 The virgin and brigand is a good first fantasy for couples. It's easy to make it an extension of her being the meek female and him being the rampaging male.

2 Teacher and pupil is another fantasy that couples often find easily acceptable. In this scenario, one partner attempts to teach, while the other deliberately makes mistakes and is sexually "punished".

3 Nurse and patient – many people get incredibly turned on seeing their partner in uniform. You can expect it to do more for him than for her.

4 Slave and mistress – not all domination games have the woman as victim. He can take a turn in being the slave and accept his due chastisement.

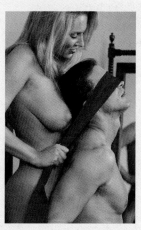

Putting on a show

Visual stimulation is very important to a man's arousal. No one expects an "amateur" stripper to be as good as a professional but it's worth practising in front of the mirror to help improve your undressing technique. Before you begin your striptease, ensure that the lighting is soft and moody and the room is warm. Use "bump and grind" music to enhance your performance. If you are wearing stockings and heels, consider leaving them on for as long as possible.

Mirrors placed at strategic points around your room of love can be used for special scenarios of exhibitionism and voyeurism. These always add a certain frisson to sexual proceedings. Your sexual "acting" in front of them can evolve naturally.

Reading out loud

Although men tend to respond to sexy photographs and high-action literature, many women freeze when they come across hard-core porn. But if you give them something suggestive to read, you can suddenly generate powerful sexual excitement. This is why one of the best things men can do in bed with women is read out loud to them.

So, for a memorable sexual experience, shut yourself up one cosy winter's afternoon with your partner. Take a seat in front of a roaring log fire, with drapes drawn against the cold and the dark. Having equipped yourself with a sexy book, let the reading session begin! Linger lovingly over the erotic paragraphs. Sexy authors may be found on the Internet by typing "erotica" into the search engine.

Mirror scenarios

Using mirrors can add excitement to your lovemaking in all sorts of ways – seeing yourself and your partner in imaginative sexual positions can be highly arousing. Find out for yourself:

1 You might pretend that the mirror is a window into the room next door. In that room, there are two lovers who are performing specially for you.
2 You might angle your lovemaking so that you can actually see the penis moving in and out of the vagina. The reflection in the mirror becomes a kind of porn movie. You might position yourself right in front of the mirror so that watching yourself becomes part of a game of submission and domination.
3 One of you might order the other to do something specifically sexual that they may never have viewed before. This might be the act of fellatio or cunnilingus, or having sex on a chair in front of the mirror.
4 Your lover might tell you that it is your job to turn him or her on. You could do this by stimulating yourself while your partner is watching you in the reflection.
5 Your lover might assist you by masturbating as he or she becomes increasingly aroused by your reflected activities.

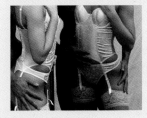

Submission and domination

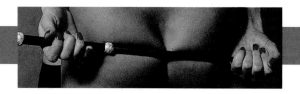

Many men and women love playing sex games of domination and submission – they enjoy **role-playing** and letting their **sexual fantasies** come to life. Couples who enjoy **sex games** are often happy to take turns being the **dominant** or **submissive** party. The list of sub/dom role-plays, such as client and **dominatrix**, is as long as your imagination. But, whatever the scenario, the games should be **highly arousing** to both parties and should **promote trust**.

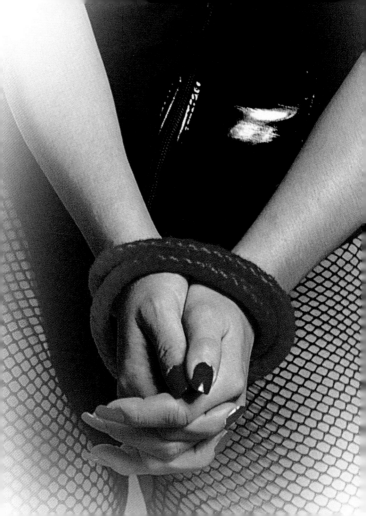

Bondage

This is the sensual art of tying up your partner to render him or her helpless. Once he or she is secured, it is the dominator or dominatrix who then tickles and teases the victim into erotic submission. So what is the attraction of bondage?

Some people need to feel securely contained: they find it very hard to "let go" enough to enjoy sexuality, but if they are rendered helpless then there's nothing they can do to prevent erotic stimulation. The constraint somehow makes it okay to experience pleasure.

Alternatively, some men and women have explored many other aspects of sexuality and no longer get the same thrill as they did at the beginning of their sex lives. Games of domination and submission may be seen as a new direction to explore and can help re-arouse slumbering sexual imaginations.

Many people are afraid of the idea of bondage, fearing that by putting themselves so utterly at someone's mercy they might be seriously harmed. If you were to practise bondage with a complete stranger, a degree of risk would certainly be involved. However, if you are in a close relationship there should be nothing to fear. It is necessary to have complete trust in a partner to be able to "let go". And before you can develop such trust, you usually have to establish a good relationship first. So it's for this reason that most bondage fans will tell you that their relationships are more open and more trusting than most others.

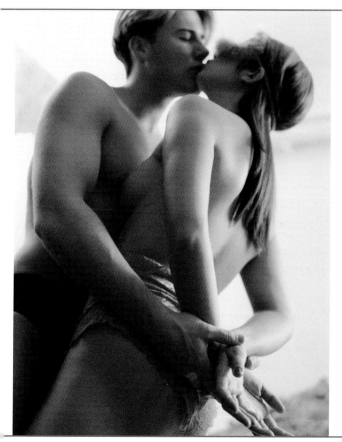

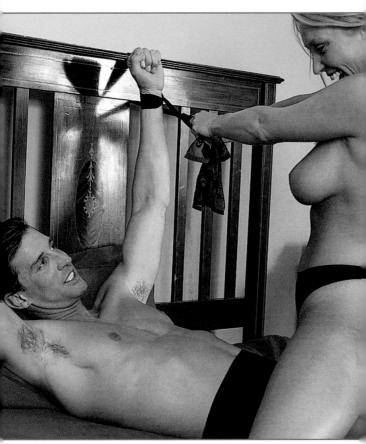

Sex slave game

Blindfold your partner and tie his or her wrists to a piece of furniture, such as a bed post. Tell your partner that he or she will now be the sexual slave of you and another person and must be ready to obey every instruction. There is no other person present in the room, but its your job to convince your partner that there is. Disguise your voice, change the way you walk and move, and vary your usual sexual techniques. Try using sex toys (see pp.136–43), such as vibrators and dildos – anything that is safe to use. Meanwhile, your partner cannot see who is performing the sexual acts on him or her – the imagination is free to run wild!

Laying down the boundaries

Talk to your partner about what is and isn't acceptable before you get to tying each other up. Agree that one of you is in charge and the other is passive, because bondage doesn't work if you are both striving to be the dominant one. The person who is in charge should also agree to stay "in character" and persevere despite "protests" from the other partner.

Agree on a code word. This is so that when your partner shouts "stop it", you know that you can carry on. But when he or she shouts the code word, you know your partner is serious and that you must stop. And if you have even the mildest suspicion that your partner may not play by the rules, do not even start this activity.

More bondage games

If your partner is keen to join you in a bondage game, you might start off with mild sexual roleplay. If, on the other hand, he or she is clearly unwilling to be tied up, do not insist they go against their inner wishes or force them. Your roleplay doesn't need to include bondage at all.

It could be as simple as the seducer having his or her wicked way with the virgin. But with follow-up lovemaking, you might continue with a slave and sultan scenario where the sultan strongly believes in the helpless passivity of his harem concubines! In other words, build up to the stronger scenarios slowly. That way, you can find out whether you both enjoy the experience, but you can still back out if necessary. Also, make sure you take it in turns to play different roles. When it comes to bondage itself, as long as you and your partner both agree to take part in a particular sex act, you both respect each other's wishes, and there is no other person involved, you are hurting no one. You could tie your partner to the bed with silken cords and tantalize him or her to climax. Alternatively, you could give your partner rules and punish him or her for breaking them – this might involve a light caning. To make the game more fun, choose rules that will be difficult to stick to.

Warning

In many countries, sexual activities that involve physically hurting others are illegal, even if they are between consenting adults.

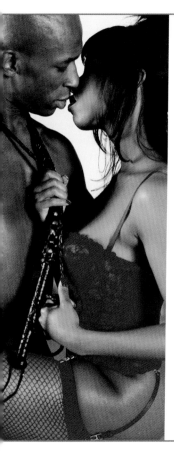

Tantalizing your partner

The aim of many sub/dom games is to stir your partner's X-rated imagination, and to frustrate him or her by tantalizing and teasing as much as giving satisfaction. What's the reasoning behind frustrating your partner? Because not being able to have what you desire arouses many people, and this increases the degree of sexual turn-on.

There are a variety of bondage props you can choose from, such as silken scarves, ties, and haberdashery-style ropes. There are commercial bondage kits consisting of specially designed couches where you can be tied up with your body at the ultimate angle for stimulation and penetration; special "swings" to strap yourself into; and even sets of "love stirrups" to wear during intercourse.

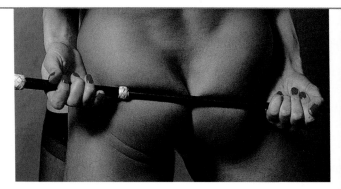

Spanking and caning

Caning and spanking may sound like painful experiences to some but, to many people, a light slap of the hand or a playful tap with a cane brings the blood pleasantly to the surface. The tingling and warming of the skin are all precursors of erotic arousal, and this degree of spanking or caning stings, but does not hurt. If you are spanking, remove rings from your fingers first. If you are tempted to cane lightly, try the instrument out on your own hand first. And when you know just how much of a sting it provides, think carefully.

Work out what your partner wants to take in the way of punishment. Do not impose your own ideas. And if your administrations begin to cause pain, call a halt. Pretend pain is one thing, real torture is totally unacceptable.

Spanking games

Safe spanking instruments include carpet beaters, soft flails, paddles, and spatulas. If used properly, these objects do not hurt. However, crops, rulers, and canes do hurt and should be used carefully. Here are some games to try:

"Say thank you"
• Every time you paddle your lover he or she must say "thank you".
• If your partner forgets to thank you, probably owing to the eroticism of the spanking, he or she must be "penalized" by another stroke.
• If your partner doesn't sound enthusiastic enough, you can increase the punishment.

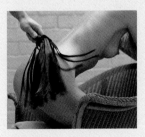

• If your partner sounds too enthusiastic, punish him or her for over-doing it.
• Make your partner count the strokes but then insist that he or she has got it wrong – even (especially) when this isn't the case.

"Where would you like it?"
• You offer your partner light spanking or caning – whichever would be most acceptable to him or her.
• You ask, "Where would you like it? Here or there?" When your partner says, "Here," then spank or cane somewhere else.
• When your partner protests, do it somewhere else again. The idea is to tease and tantalize, although sometimes you will spank in the desired place.

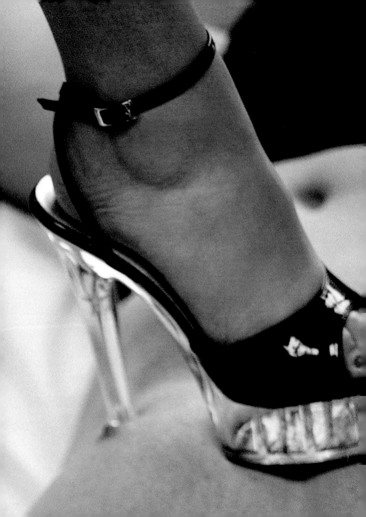

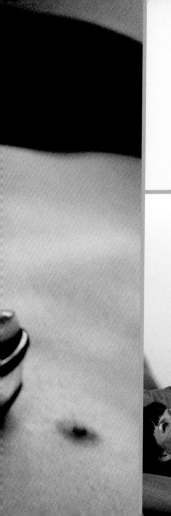

4

Sex
extras

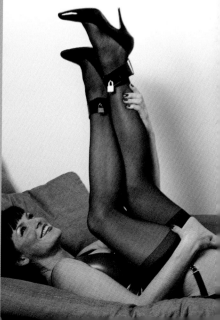

Bedroom toys

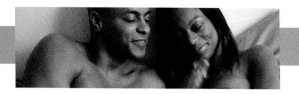

Most of the **best sex** games use props and other items to **extend and enhance** the action. If straight sex is your favourite, then a **vibrator** still manages to add to the **excitement**. If something darker gets your **pulse racing**, look to blindfolds, restraints, and a variety of other sex toys to **extend** your experience of sensuality.

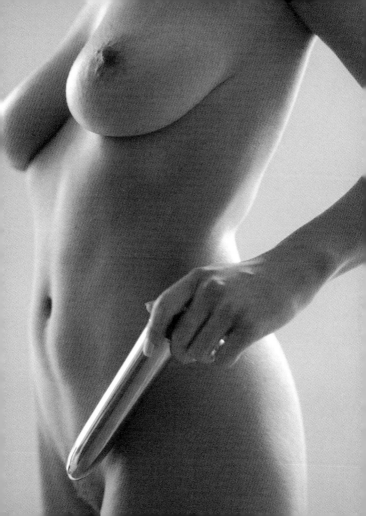

Vibrators

There's a small revolution going on in the sex-toys industry. Although the old-fashioned, hard, penis-shaped vibrators are still available, manufacturers have been concentrating on improving the design and texture of vibrators. Many are made from exciting new materials – some are soft and malleable, feeling like real skin, and there are those made from a translucent, jelly-feel substance. Some are gorgeous and jewel-like in colour.

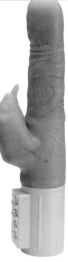

Dual-action vibrators
These feature a shaft for penetration plus a "finger" to stimulate the clitoris.

Another fantastic feature of modern vibrators is that they tend to be a lot quieter than they used to be. Vibrator designers are beginning to think seriously (and creatively) about the acts that men and women actually want their vibrators for. The result of this is a variety of very distinct shapes that are intended to carry out specific tasks. One of the most popular designs, a dual-action model, vibrates the clitoris while simultaneously probing the vagina or anus. Another new innovation is the pulsating vibrator, pulsation for some

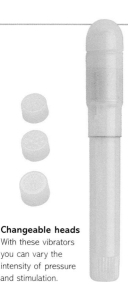

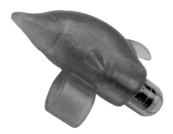

Changeable heads

With these vibrators you can vary the intensity of pressure and stimulation.

Small and discreet

This dolphin-shaped vibrator slips over a finger and needs only one tiny battery. It is water-proof, so is ideal for sex in the shower.

women being integral to their orgasm, especially for G-spot stimulation. It comes with a variable speed and throb dial.

For women who have difficulty climaxing during intercourse, there's a strap-on model that's held in place over the clitoris to provide extra stimulation while the man penetrates the vagina. The tiny finger vibrator is one of the most ingenious of the new sex toys. It's good for surprises during intercourse, since it's virtually undetectable. Some kits include textured rubber pads for varying finger sensation.

Dildos

Penis-substitutes, or dildos, have been used as sex toys since time immemorial. They are non-vibrating, and are designed for vaginal or anal penetration (or sometimes both at the same time) by women or men.

Today, dildos are usually made of latex or silicone. They may be held in the hand, or some can be slipped into a harness that is worn around the hips. The benefit of this is that the wearer keeps his or her hands free for other stimulating activity. Some models fit into a vibrating cock ring, which provides clitoral stimulation at the same time.

There are also double dildos available, which work in a push-pull fashion, and enable you and your partner to enjoy vaginal or anal penetration simultaneously.

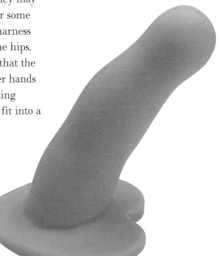

The flared base of this dildo makes it ideal for slipping into a harness to create a strap-on (see facing page). The dildo could also be used by hand.

140

Cock rings

The cock ring fits around the base of the penis. Its tight grip restricts blood from flowing back out of the penis, thus strengthening the erection and giving a feeling of fullness and pressure. It is especially useful for men who suffer from venous leakage problems. The more fun versions vibrate, and have various bumps and protrusions on them to stimulate the clitoris during intercourse.

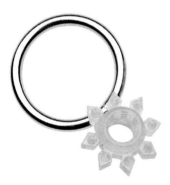

Cock rings come in many shapes and sizes, from the basic remedial penis ring to the knobbly, jelly-like clitoral tickler.

Fun lubes

Lubes enable wonderful, warm, slippery sex, and are a great help for some women at certain "dry" times of the month. They are also essential for all anal play, since the anus doesn't provide a natural lubricant. Lubes come in all colours, textures, and scents. For sheer variety, you might consider edible lubes, which are small, gelatine-filled capsules that you bite on during oral sex to flood your partner's genitals with sweet-smelling, edible gel (chocolate flavour is a popular choice). Some of the best-equipped bedrooms display rows of little gelatine pots to choose from.

Anal wands

Several vibrators are specially designed to penetrate the anus comfortably and massage the super-sensitive prostate gland situated at the far end (see p.197). This gland, which exists primarily for the purpose of manufacturing semen, is so sensitive that only brief massage can trigger climax. The anal wand is ideal for those who like a feeling of pressure combined with vibration and movement. Vibrating anal toys help relax the anal muscles if tense, and can be immensely pleasurable.

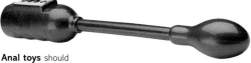

Anal toys should have a large or flared base to prevent them from slipping inside and getting lost. This sizable wand, with speed adjustments on the handle, is easily long enough to reach the prostate gland.

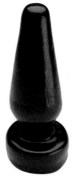

Butt plugs

Butt plugs are used in the anus or vagina, and are designed to be worn for a feeling of fullness. They are made in silicone or rubber, and are available in a variety of shapes and sizes. There is a long, thin, pointed plug (see left), a shorter, fatter, slightly curved version, and a small, squat, beaded version.

Electrical toys

Many of you will have heard of TENS machines. These are used in physiotherapy to relieve pain, and work by pulsating a tiny electrical charge into the skin. Now there's a sexual version – a wand that, when held near your body, bombards you with a continuous stream of safe, low-voltage, mini-lightning bolts. The sensations are fantastic.

Blindfolds and restraints

A blindfold offers a sense of helplessness, and makes you feel vulnerable. You don't know where you are when you wear it, and you have no idea what obstacles you may be facing. Your mind starts racing as you imagine the hazards that lie outside, and your anxiety levels being to rise. It's these swirling emotions that the astute partner tunes into and utilizes – generally, the greater the anxiety level, the more intense are the emotions involved.

Most games of restraint involve one partner wearing a blindfold. For comfort, use a soft material such as a silk scarf, a black velvet eye mask, or a sleep mask. Make sure that you don't tie the blindfold too tight, which could be painful, or too loosely, unless partial sight is intended as part of a game. Unless you know that your partner is into really serious bondage, it's best to use restraints made of soft fabrics, such as a man's silky tie, or the silky cord from a dressing gown. Alternatively, most of the sex-toy manufacturers sell "safe" handcuffs, specially designed for the purpose of sex-play.

Sex boosters

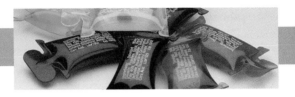

There are numerous ways of giving your sex life a boost. Using your **imagination** is **paramount,** but the sex-toy industry and drug companies have developed an **increasing range** of products designed to help **reduce inhibition** and **enhance sexual response.**

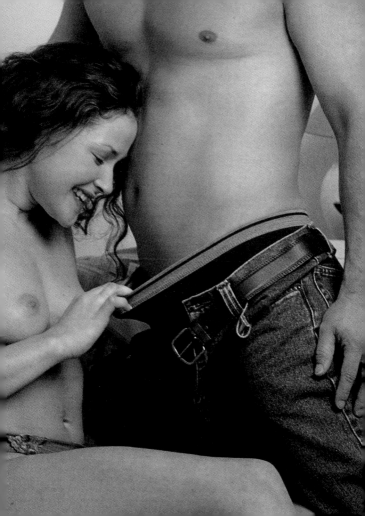

Books and magazines

There is no doubt that men are turned on by sexy pictures of women, and sex tests have shown that men are also frequently turned on by hard porn. Women, on the other hand, tend to be aroused by suggestive, less overtly sexual literature, and generally don't find visual images as exciting.

These sex tests seem to have pointed to an innate sex difference between men and women. But whatever your preference for pictures or words, the imagination is one of the biggest sex enhancers of all, and erotic books and magazines act as an excellent starting point for the imagination.

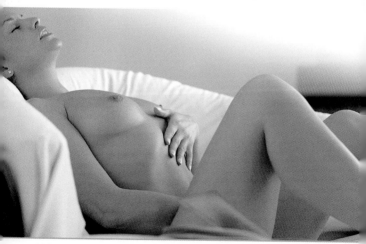

Erotic clothing

Dressing up can act as an extremely exciting forerunner to an erotic encounter. In addition to sexy underwear, shoes, and stockings, there is now a wide range of outfits available in sensual fabrics, such as PVC and shiny rubber. These hug every crevice of the wearer's body and feel amazingly sexy; they will also drive your partner mad with desire.

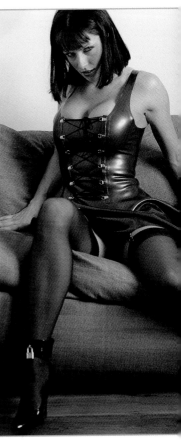

Powerful boosters

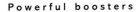

A study where single women were given testosterone replacement therapy showed that several dropped out, finding themselves unable to cope with their increased sexual desire levels.

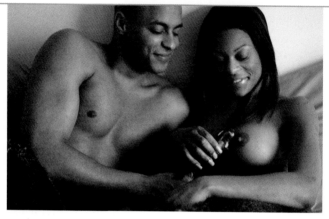

Sex toys

The sex-toy industry is increasingly developing new products for both sexes, but particularly for women. This is because a revolution has gone on in the bedroom enabling women to become more overtly sexual – like men, they want to overcome inhibitions and enjoy sex, and welcome any product that allows them to do so in the easiest possible way. Sex tool products range from new and exciting vibrators, specially designed to suit women's eroticism and sensibilities, as well as anal wands and other products aimed at men.

Some sex toys work by pulsating an electrical charge into the skin, producing an incredible array of sensations.

Reducing inhibitions

A couple of glasses of wine can improve your love life because the alcohol relaxes you while lowering your inhibitions, and this lets your naturally sexy, raunchy side emerge. But if you drink more than two glasses, it can begin to have the opposite effect: it can depress sex drive, and make you feel sleepy and uncoordinated. In men, it can lead to "brewer's droop", where it becomes difficult to maintain an erection.

Sex doctors now know that the pharmaceutical drug phentolamine works on the "inhibitor" brain centre by loosening up a person's inhibitions and allowing sexual desire to come to the surface, where previously it may have been repressed. This drug is available by prescription only.

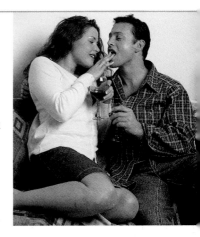

Poppers

Poppers are capsules containing the drug amyl nitrate. If the drug is sniffed shortly before orgasm, it lowers the blood pressure, slows the heart up, and slows down the sensation of orgasm.

WARNING: The use of poppers can cause headaches, nausea, and disorientation. They are unsafe if they are taken in conjunction with Viagra.

Viagra and viacreme

A small revolution occurred with the recent development of Viagra, which provides impotent men with a good erection. The beauty of Viagra is that it can only function when the brain thinks sexy thoughts, so it does not reduce stimulation to a purely mechanical act.

The drug works by boosting the nitric oxide level in the region of the genitals, allowing erections to be sustained. Some women find their sexual response is improved by taking Viagra, but since the drug was designed for men, it is not advisable for women to take it. Viacreme is a cream that can be rubbed on to the clitoris or penis. It draws the blood to your genitals, and helps trigger the start of your erection (or the female equivalent). See the Internet for more details.

Viacreme
Your partner can apply this to your penis or clitoris during foreplay. You will soon start to feel a sexy, tingling sensation.

Testosterone

The hormone testosterone is a strong chemical component of male physiological make up. However, a few men have a testosterone deficiency, which is sometimes associated with the andropause – these men could perk up their sex lives if they took testosterone supplements. Similarly, women who find it difficult to experience orgasm should get a blood test to check their testosterone levels. If these are low, testosterone therapy may help to improve their sexual response.

Testosterone is available in gel form. Since there are health implications to taking it, it is wise to see a doctor and get it on prescription. However, many doctors are still unfamiliar with testosterone replacement therapy. The gel is also available on the Internet.

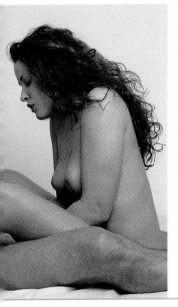

Dressing for sex

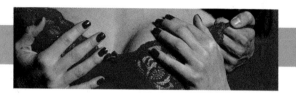

When dressing for sex, the rules are simple: wear **tight clothes** that **emphasize** the **curves** and **contours** of the body and draw the eye to the genitals, chest, or buttocks. Clothes should either be difficult to take off, the idea being that you **tease your partner** into submission while remaining inaccessible, or extremely **easy to slip out of**.

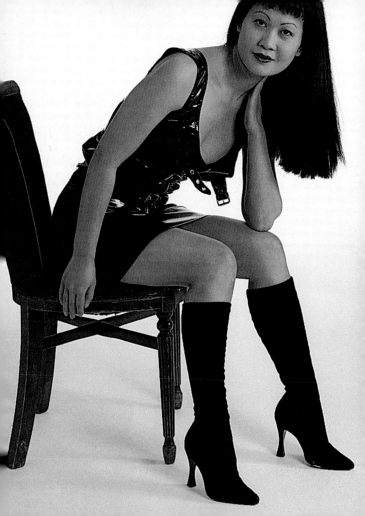

Choosing underwear

Because underwear is the last item of clothing that you shed before sex, it has an important symbolic value. When that underwear is silky and sexy, it can have a wonderfully sensual effect, making you feel great and your partner long to get his or her hands on you. Men have fewer types of underwear to choose from but, rather than get complacent about your choice, buy something that you know your partner finds attractive

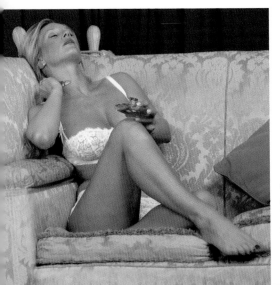

Your choice of underwear can help you play a sexual role. White underwear conjures up ideas of virginity.

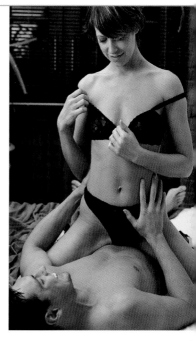

— black silk boxers are often popular. If you don't know what he or she likes, try drawing up a humorous list with your partner, covering the types of underwear that you find sexy and those that you dislike.

Take each other's vital measurements, and then go shopping together. Let sexual tension start in the underwear department and build on the way home. Some sex shops specialize solely in erotic underwear, from crotchless panties and G-strings to leather and rubber ware. You can even buy edible underwear.

When undressing each other, try a game of removing each other's underwear with your teeth — the only thing that you're allowed to use your hands for is her bra clip.

Use underwear as a sexual shorthand to tell your partner what kind of sex to expect — black, lacy underwear expresses confidence and sexual assurance, and shows your man that you want to take control.

Shoes

For years the foot, and its clothing – the shoe – have been seen as an erotic symbol of the female body. Indeed, there were generations of men who equated a dainty foot with powerful sex appeal. But that was back in the days when nice women didn't show their legs.

Today, we are not focused on the foot in quite the same way. However, if you plant a tall, slim woman, wearing sheer black stockings, a short skirt, and tremendously high stiletto heels in front of a male you will see a fascinating phenomenon – presented with such a vision of a long-legged woman, men virtually froth at the mouth. Today's psychologists believe that this is a result of males becoming fixated as children on particular sights or objects that they accidentally associate with sexuality.

Out of this, a thriving industry of high-heeled shoes has grown – these used to be called tart's shoes because prostitutes were so aware of their pulling power. Seamed stockings and high black leather boots also dramatically outline and draw attention to a sexy leg.

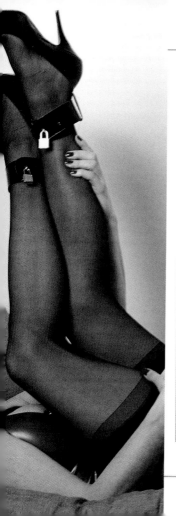

Erotic foot

Feet have long been associated with sex – in both men and women, toes tend to curl involuntarily during orgasm. In fact, the feet are so rich in nerve endings that some people are able to climax from foot caresses alone.

In literature, the foot has been used to symbolize the female genitals – for example, the story of Cinderella can be read as a story about sexual fit. And in Japanese erotic art, curled toes have been stylized symbols of erotic response for hundreds of years.

There is a form of lovemaking called pedic lovemaking. This includes the man having his penis massaged by the woman's feet. It also includes sucking the toes of a female partner, using the big toe to stimulate the clitoris or vagina. Many women enjoy having their feet held and caressed during sexual intercourse. Experiment with these techniques with your partner to see if they have the desired effect.

Throw a party

You and your partner could organize a fancy dress party – the condition of entry is that guests must dress as their favourite sexual fetish or fantasy:

1 Tight leather – anything made of leather has sadomasochistic overtones, especially when belts and chains are added.
2 Fake fur – this suggests decadence, especially if you are completely naked beneath a fake fur coat.
3 Tribal and ethnic clothes – exotic clothing from foreign cultures can be flattering and suggestive. Wear saris, sarongs, grass skirts, bikinis made of flowers, feathers, or veils. You could also dress up as a belly- or limbo dancer.
4 Uniforms – symbols of authority are always sexy. Dress up as a policeman, fireman, doctor, nurse, or teacher. Alternatively, servant and schoolgirl uniforms suggest

servility and innocence.
5 Cross-dressing – try to create at least a moment's uncertainty when you make your entrance as to your true gender.

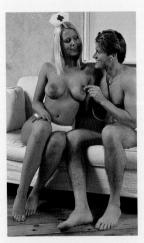

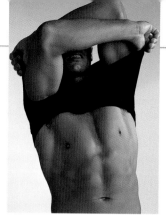

Body adornments

Body piercing and tattoos used to be regarded as a very primitive and even mutilating form of art. Indeed, there are many people who still see them like this and dislike the look of them. But in the past five years a new middle-class phenomenon has grown up, mainly among the younger generation. Many young men and women sprout a plethora of earrings, nose rings, and body jewelry with pride.

Piercing and tattoos are often a means of a young person distinguishing him or herself from parents or other members of the older generation. They can be a statement of independence and confidence. There is also a sense of taking part in a rite of passage — couples or friends go to the tattooist or piercer together.

Sexy undressing

If you're not used to stripping, the following exercise can help. Stand in front of a full-length mirror, pretend that you're alone, and very slowly take off all of your clothes. Take time to really look at your body in the mirror and touch yourself in whatever way you want to. This takes away the performance aspect of stripping and gives your partner the sense of being a voyeur. If it makes you feel better, let your partner hide in the next room and watch you from behind the door.

It's no accident that both being pierced and being tattooed involve a certain amount of pain. Yet both experiences are regularly described as erotic.

Certain people associate the pain of skin piercing with the pleasure of sexual arousal. And piercings, through the nipples and genitals, are associated with the sex act.

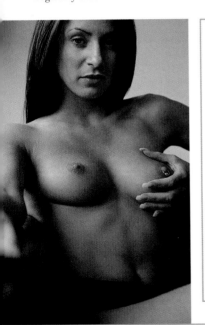

Safe piercing

Ensure that the metal used in your piercing jewelry is surgical steel, gold, or platinum, and be scrupulous about aftercare – poor hygiene can cause an unsightly infection.

Generally safe places to pierce are the belly button, eyebrow, ears and nose. Less safe places to pierce are the tongue (takes enamel off the teeth); lips (might get wrenched when kissing or wiping mouth); nipples (might impair female's breast-feeding in the future); and genitals (damp, moist area might lead to infection).

Wearers of body jewelry say that their piercings give them extra arousal and make the visual side of intercourse – such as hardened nipples – powerfully erotic.

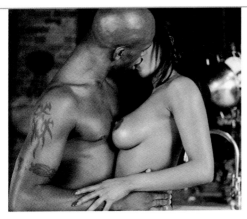

Tattoos give the impression of strength and confidence, which can be very attractive to others. They can relate specifically to a lover, such as a name, and can be an indelible statement of enduring love.

Considering tattoos

Hidden tattoos, on the inner arms, thighs, and buttocks can be sexy discoveries for lovers to make. Even the genitals can be tattooed. However, a permanent tattoo is a major commitment – once the skin has been injected with indelible dye, you gain a body adornment that lasts for a lifetime. Always consider carefully where a tattoo will be positioned, and what it will show because whatever you choose will be with you through your life, and you don't want to grow tired of it. It is probably best to experiment first with henna tattoos that last for a few days and can be removed with oil. You can even have temporary tattoos custom-made, which may be a preferable option.

Sensual materials

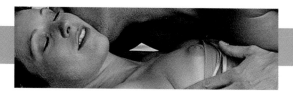

When **venturing** into the world of **exotic sex**, among the first delights to incorporate into your love life are **sensual props**. If you've never experienced the teasing of velvet or the slither of silk across your skin, you can now anticipate a range of **exquisite sensations**.

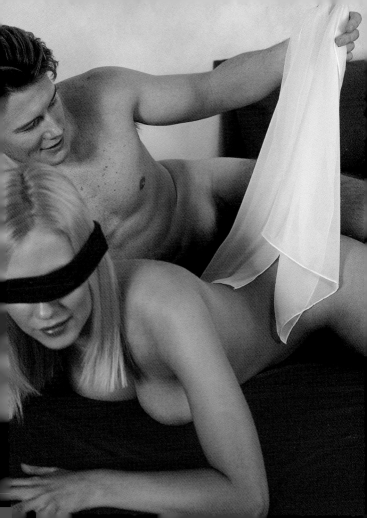

Pleasing the senses

Set time aside for the two of you to indulge in a really sensuous evening. Equip yourselves with squares of sensual fabrics, such as silk, velvet, and fur. Using a long strand of velvet, blindfold your partner and lead him or her into an excessively heated room.

Make sure that the room is already scented with perfume or a burning, sweet-smelling joss stick. As your partner stands there blindfolded, say that he or she must submit to anything you choose to do. This is the cue to slowly peel off your lover's clothes and lay him or her on a spacious sofa or a bed covered by a large piece of velvet.

Tell your partner it is imperative that he or she lies there with legs apart. Now is the cue to stroke every inch of his or her skin with each of your

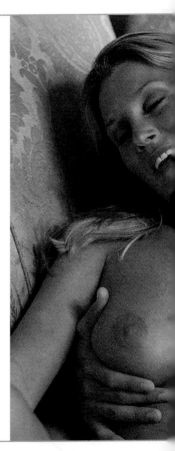

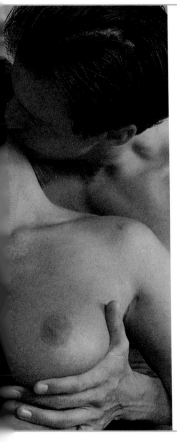

sensual fabrics. You can whisk them across the main part of the body, use them to tickle and tease, and use the materials to massage the body with, avoiding the genitals at this stage.

Throughout this experience, your partner will be wondering what is going to happen between the legs. Keep your lover waiting for as long as possible: the anticipation will heighten the pleasure. Not until you have thoroughly pleasured the rest of the body do you then repeat the process with the genitals.

Sumptuous fabrics

Lying naked on sumptuous furnishing fabrics adds to feelings of anticipation and excitement and soft, light fabrics, such as silks and satins, can be run along your partner's body to tease and tempt.

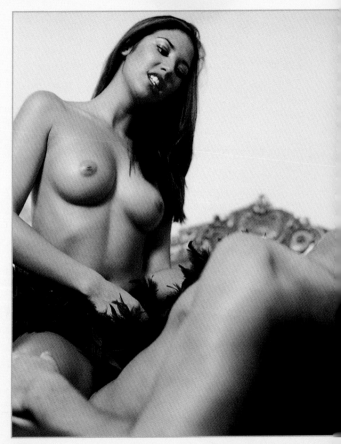

Teasing with feathers

One of the most exotic touch temptations is the feather massage, which you could use as a preliminary to a sensual or genital massage. Feathers look gorgeous, skim lightly across the skin, and tickle the innocent recipient into wriggling submission. You could use a feather boa, or a single peacock feather for more directed sensation in this teasing routine:

1 Tickle every single inch of your partner's skin with either the feather boa or peacock feather, using light, rapid movements.

2 Sprinkle your partner with talc and use the boa or plume to sweep the powder across their body in long, even strokes.

3 Sweep the boa or plume from the knees upwards along your partner's inside thigh, "accidentally" touching the genitals when you reach the tops of the legs.

Top materials

Certain materials have extremely sensual or suggestive textures:
• Velvet
• Satin
• Silk
• Feathers
• Fur
• Leather
• Rubber
• PVC
• Clingfilm
• Canvas (harness, straps)

Fetishes

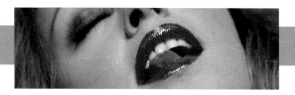

Fetishists are people who are **sexually stimulated** by a **particular object**, and whose fetishes do not conform to heterosexual or homosexual sex. While many people possess minor **fetishes** that have no great impact on their sex lives, major **sexual variations** inevitably influence relationships.

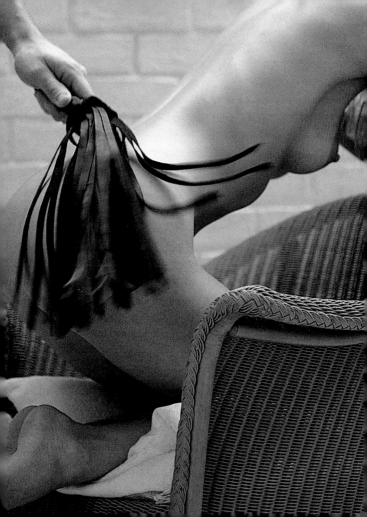

Fetish theories

According to the theories, the fetishist (usually male) is often extremely introverted and anxious about forming relationships. Afraid of rejection, he unconsciously attaches himself to something inanimate or partial that could not reject him. As a child, he may have associated an object with the stirrings of sexual arousal and may subconsciously "remember" this the next time he sees the object or feels sexy. The two memories become irrevocably linked, and the fetish is born.

It doesn't necessarily have to be sexual arousal that causes sexual associations – in situations where adrenaline (the "fight and flight" hormone) is aroused, people are put into a state of extra awareness. In 1980, psychologists Chris Gosselin and Glenn Wilson made a study of "rubberites", particularly rubber mackintosh enthusiasts. Most of their subjects felt that their interest had developed in their childhood, during World War II. Gosselin and Wilson surmised that the anxiety-provoking circumstances of war, plus a lot of rubber articles in use at the time, provided fertile ground for this particular interest.

Learning theorists argue that individuals can virtually programme themselves to become fetishists by association.

Warning

If you do not want to take part in a certain sexual activity, do not hesitate to say no. No one should be forced to have sex that is repugnant to them.

Women and fetishes

Very few women are fetishists. This is probably because many girls, unlike boys, often don't discover their sexual response until their late teenage years or even their twenties, by which time they have learned to associate sex with a relationship rather than an attraction to specific parts of the body or even objects. Women fetishists often (but not always) associate their special sexual interests with some kind of emotional wounding.

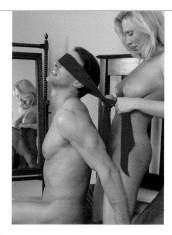

Visual-mental link

Dr. Glenn Wilson of the Institute of Psychiatry (UK) believes that the area in the male brain which is responsible for male sexuality is situated extremely close to the area that is responsible for seeing. This may account for the theory that men are more turned on by visual stimuli than women, and that experiences can "leak" from one section of the brain to the other.

Fetish and philia glossary

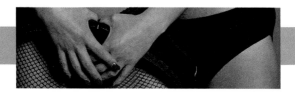

Virtually anything can become a **fetish**, although fetishes **change with the times** and fashions. In the 19th century, for example, when **ladies wore gloves**, hand fetishes were common. Today, this fetish has all but disappeared. Over the past 50 years or so, new fetishes for modern, **man-made fabrics,** such as **PVC**, have emerged. This section features the **most common** fetishes.

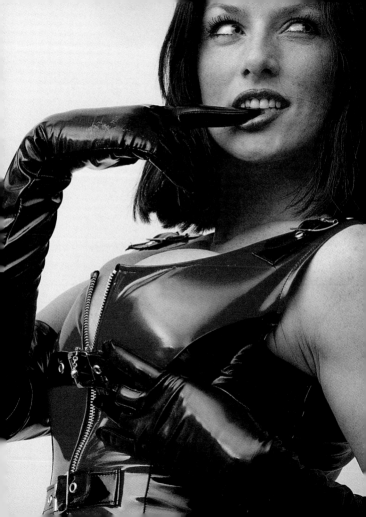

Amputee fetish

Some people (usually men) are sexually stimulated by people who are missing certain limbs. The theory behind this attraction is that if the male fetishist feels sexually inadequate, the realization that he has a physical advantage over the disabled individual allows him to feel powerful and sexually aroused.

Autoerotic asphyxia

This is a highly dangerous activity in which a male or female restricts their breathing in order to accentuate or prolong the experience of orgasm, often by hanging themselves by the neck or putting a plastic bag over the head. This lowers oxygen and blood pressure, and increases carbon dioxide intake. Don't do it!

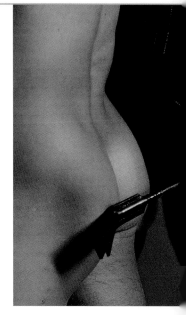

Bondage

An activity where a dominant partner binds a submissive one so that they cannot escape (see pp.124–133). A major effect of bondage is the release of normal

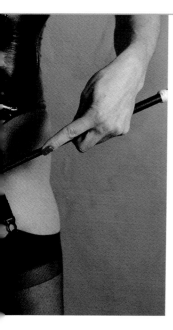

Cinderella fetish (Podophilia)

One of the most common fetishes among both men and women, this is a passion for shoes. Imelda Marcos of the Philippines possessed rooms full of shoes – we don't know if she derived sexual pleasure from them, but there must have been some special emotion here in order to collect so many pairs so avidly. (See also High-heel fetish, p.177)

Defilement fetish

Some fetishists get very turned-on by looking at other people covered in mud, slime, and other messy substances.

Exhibitionism

Some men and women get a major frisson from knowing they might be observed doing

inhibitions on the grounds that there is nothing the submissive partner can do to prevent the activity. (See also string or clingfilm bondage, p.180)

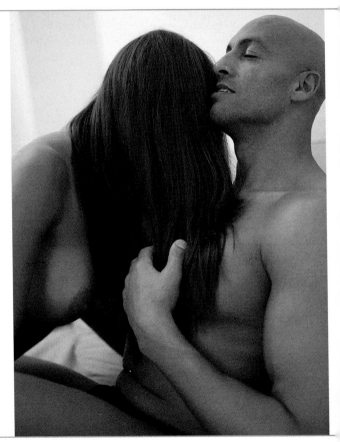

something sexual. Sex outdoors with the chance of being seen, for example, is particularly attractive to many individuals.

Frottage

The activity of rubbing genitals against someone's body in order to arouse sexual excitement is attractive to many people. It can be done during sexual intercourse but also, more sinisterly, in public places to strangers, such as on a crowded train.

Golden showers (Urolagnia)

Many people find urinating on their partner or being urinated on enhances sexual pleasure, relishing the warmth and the mess involved. Couples spray "golden rain" onto the face, body, or genitals of a partner, often during sex or while bathing or showering.

Hair fetish (Trichophilia)

An obsession with hair sometimes leads to hair fetishists creeping up behind strangers in the street or on public transport and snipping off their locks.

High-heel fetish (Altocalciphilia)

This is an advanced form of the Cinderella fetish (see p.175), where the male enthusiast gets carried away by the sight of women's high-heeled shoes. This fascination probably develops when the fetishist is a young boy and when unconsciously he sees high heels looming over him and accidentally associates the sight with sexual sensation.

Infantilism

A sex game, usually played by fairly powerful men, which involves being looked after like a baby. Infantilism fetishists enjoy being dressed in baby clothes, especially nappies, given bottles of milk to drink, and having their nappies changed. The final touch to the game would be stimulation by "nanny" to orgasm, although not all men want to go that far. The common explanation for this fetish is that powerful men with a lot of responsibility sometimes need to feel totally helpless and without responsibility of any sort. There are weekend breaks on offer, where business men can go to be "nannied".

Kokigami

A Japanese enthusiasm, where the male wraps his penis in a paper costume (the name means origami of the penis). This idea originated in Japan in the 8th century, when aristocrats wrapped their genitals in silky trimmings and then offered them as gifts to their lovers, enjoying the sensual experience of them being unwrapped.

Mud-wrestling fetish

See Defilement fetish, p.175.

Necrophilia

Literally speaking, this means making love to a corpse, and no doubt there are some disturbed individuals who do just that. But it can also refer to the practice of making love to a victim who plays dead, lying totally inert, regardless of what is done to him or her. The attraction for the fetishist is total control.

Pony-racing fetish

The competitive activity of "pony-racing" is an extension of sado-masochistic gaming. The "drivers" tend to be male and the "ponies", often pulling real (but lightweight) pony carts, are usually women, partially nude but bound with harness straps. Often there is an element of pain to their pulling, and the driver is likely to encourage speed by using his whip. Pony-racing clubs hold regular racing events for their members.

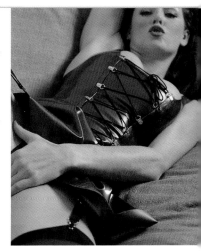

Public-speaking fetish (Homilophilia)

Some people get turned-on by standing up in front of an audience and making a sexually fuelled speech; others become excited by listening and may end up bouncing compulsively on the edge of his or her seat.

Rubber fetish

Rubber fetishists are aroused by wellington boots, rubber mackintoshes, and rubber aprons. Many wear underwear made out of latex, and costumes, such as nuns' habits, vests, skirts, and hoods, are also part of the specialist clothing on offer. Rubber sheets are also available.

String or clingfilm bondage

String bondage is a specialized form of sado-masochism, in which the submissive partner is tied up or wrapped with string around certain areas of the body. Clingfilm is a modern material used for the same effect, and can be subtly provocative. Games involve winding the wrap between a woman's legs so that her labia is trapped open under a layer of clingfilm but so that the entrance to her vagina remains unobstructed. Alternatively, a male wraps it around his scrotum to form a kind of testes ring, or around the shaft of his penis with only the head left free. An important word of caution: clingfilm must never be wrapped around the face, especially the mouth or nose.

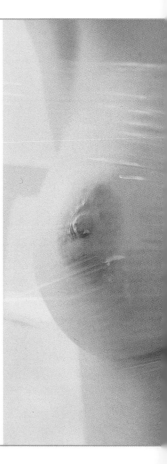

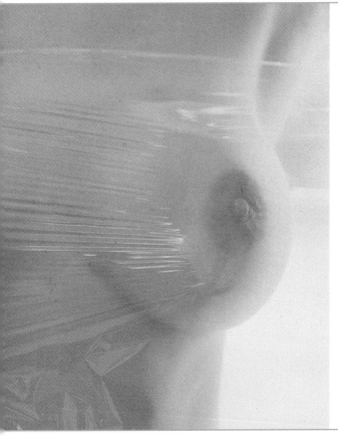

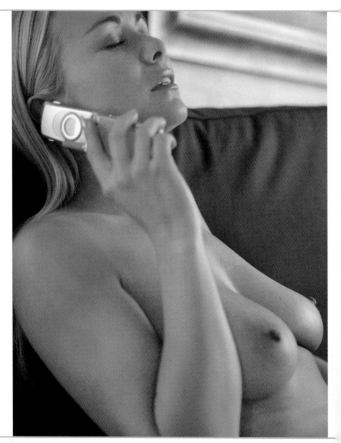

Telephonicophilia

Telephone fetishists get a thrill from calling strangers and shocking them with the use of deliberately explicit sexual conversation. Alternatively, they may be enthusiasts of telephone sex during which men and women masturbate while consciously arousing each other on the telephone.

Vampirism

This can refer to any sex play where blood is involved. Originally, the expression specifically referred to drinking blood, with Dracula as a prime example of the true vampirist. Warning: Since vampirism involves exchanging blood, it is considered to constitute unsafe sex, and you run the risk of contracting AIDS by indulging in this practice.

Voyeurism

Some people, commonly known as "Peeping Toms", get sexually aroused by watching other people engage in sexual activity. Such enthusiasts will often masturbate while watching the activity or will stimulate themselves later while they "relive" the event.

Zoophilia

This fetish overlaps with beastiality. Some people are sexually stimulated either by the thought of sex with animals or by the activity itself. Primitive societies have traditionally engaged in sex with animals when human beings are not available. Since becoming more urban, zoophilia has diminished in Western societies. Popular zoophilia subjects are dogs and horses.

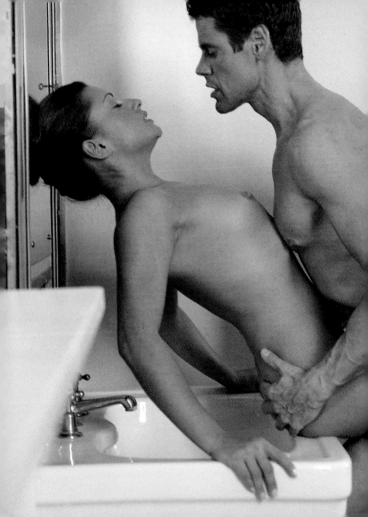

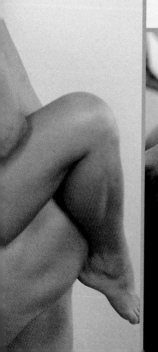
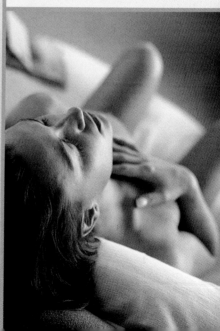

5

Orgasm
and response

Sexual response in both sexes

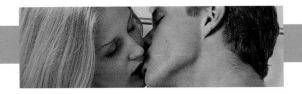

Men and women's physiological experience
of **sexual arousal** is remarkably similar. Each
undergoes at least three stages of response.
These consist of **desire**, **arousal**, and **orgasm**,
after which the body returns to its previous
unstimulated state (this is known as "**resolution**").

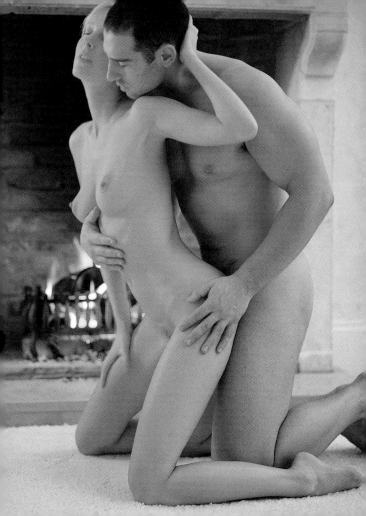

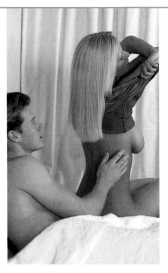

Desire

The preliminary stage of sexual response in both sexes is desire. This is when the idea of sex first comes into your head, and is usually triggered by a sexy thought or touch. In theory, it is not about the turn-on of the body although, particularly with men, the two stages (desire and arousal) can occur almost concurrently. Males are usually more turned on by a visual stimulus than females, whereas in women it is often the idea of a man – the whole person – that creates female desire.

Kaplan's theory

Dr Helen Singer Kaplan claimed that the three stages of sexual response (desire, arousal, and orgasm) were not necessarily always linked – each stage can be experienced independently of the others. For example, some women can experience desire but cannot become aroused or have an orgasm. Other women never feel desire, but do manage to get easily aroused by touch. A few women experience no desire or arousal but can have orgasms, which they may hardly feel.

Arousal

The next stage of the response cycle is arousal, where the body undergoes a series of visible changes as excitement builds. Many of these changes are common to both sexes – the blood rushes to the genitals, the body perspires, the nipples harden, and the heart rate, blood pressure, breathing rate, and muscle tension increase. The physical changes make the body extra-sensitive to touch and stimulation, increasing the participants' pleasure further.

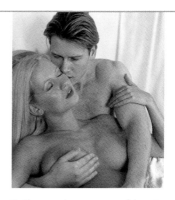

Physiological changes during arousal

As sexual excitement builds, blood pressure rises by about one-third, reaching even higher at orgasm. This rise in blood pressure is slightly greater in men than in women.

Both sexes have a normal heart rate of about 80 beats per minute (bpm). In the plateau phase, this more than doubles. At orgasm, a woman's bpm can reach 175 and a man's 180. When excited, the breathing patterns of both men and women change. They breathe much more loudly and quickly than normal. At the point of orgasm, they are taking as many as 40 breaths per minute, twice the normal number.

Timing of sexual response

Although men and women experience sexual excitement in similar ways, there are also considerable differences, particularly in the timing of the key stages of sexual response. Men tend to become aroused very quickly, and this stage is then followed by a relatively long plateau phase before orgasm. Women generally take longer to become fully aroused, and require a lot more stimulation than men to reach the same point. However, their plateau stage, between arousal and orgasm, is shorter than in men.

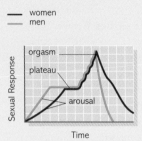

— women
— men

Extending the plateau Men tend to reach the plateau phase within a few minutes, while women need about 15–30 minutes. For this reason, a man needs to wait for his partner to catch up.

Orgasm

When sensations become increasingly intense, both partners experience a peak of pleasure called orgasm. Orgasm is similar for the sexes, containing exactly the same timing of

orgasmic contractions. With men, orgasm is almost inevitably accompanied by the ejaculation of seminal fluid. The majority of men associate climax with their genital area, and only rarely experience orgasm elsewhere. Orgasmic contractions for men and for women occur at intervals of 0.8 seconds. Women, however, appear to be capable of experiencing orgasm in many different sites of the body, including, in some cases, the entire body. Orgasms for both sexes may be long and strong, short and weak, sometimes a mere flutter, other times so drawn out that they last for almost a minute. What's more, all of these variations may be experienced by one individual during a lifetime.

Resolution

After orgasm, the body returns to its original resting state. The body tension is released, the blood flow drains from the genitals, the heart rate, blood pressure, and sex flush subside, and the breathing returns to normal. This process is usually considerably quicker for men than women, who can often remain aroused for some time after orgasm, and with continued stimulation can experience climax for a second or a third time or more.

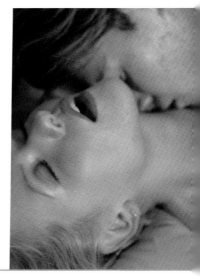

His sexual response

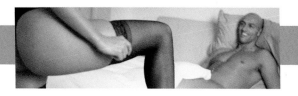

The sexual response cycle starts off with feelings of desire. This is frequently triggered by a visual stimulus – for example, the glimpse of a **woman's thigh** as she puts on her **stockings**, or **her breasts** as she fastens her bra. Alternatively, a **sexy thought** or a light touch can put ideas into a man's head. **Sexual interest** will then register in his brain, which will in turn transmit **signals** to his **genitals**. The next stage is arousal, when fairly dramatic physiological changes start to take place, then finally **orgasm**.

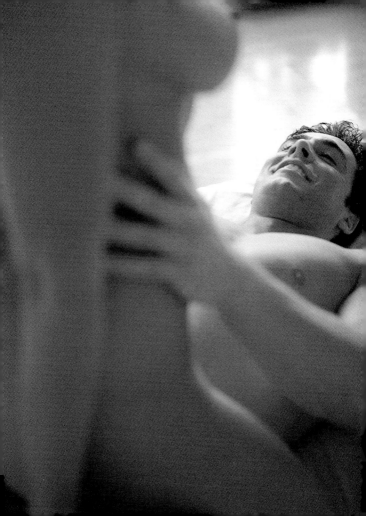

Arousal stages

Once the brain has registered sexual interest, it sends a message to the penis. In most cases, the man has an erection within seconds. When stimulated, the erect penis then sends further sensual feeling back to the brain and to other areas of the body, causing further excitement.

1 During arousal, large amounts of blood rush to the spongy tissues of the penis, making it large and stiff.

2 Before the brain registers desire, the penis hangs down in its flaccid state. (The genitals return to this state shortly after orgasm, at the stage sometimes known as "resolution".)

3 The scrotum thickens and the testicles are drawn up to the body. As more blood flows into the penis, the glans (penis head) swells further and becomes a dark red or purplish colour.

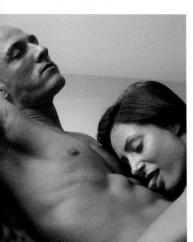

Male arousal

Men generally become sexually aroused within 10–30 seconds of initial stimulation, although this timing varies according to the individual.

All-over body changes

During sexual arousal, muscles in the body become tense, particularly at orgasm. Involuntary muscle contractions tend to cause erect nipples, arched feet, and curled toes.

At the most intense phase of sexual arousal, about 25 per cent of men show a reddening of the skin. This coloration is known as the "sex flush", and it begins on the stomach and then spreads to cover the chest, neck, and face.

Many men perspire, especially on the hands and feet but sometimes all over the body, including the neck and back.

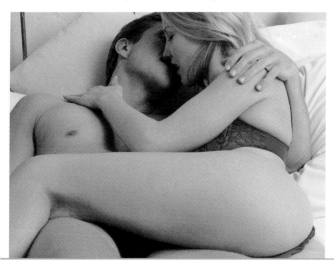

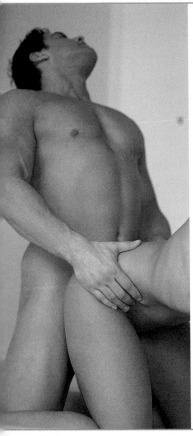

Reaching orgasm

At a high point of arousal, the tension and sensual feeling build up so intensely that orgasm is triggered, consisting of penile contractions (at approximately 0.8 second intervals) and usually resulting in ejaculation of seminal fluid. At the moment of orgasm, breathing is twice as fast as it would be normally. The heartbeat is more than double its usual rate, and blood pressure is increased by one-third.

Most men can sense when they are about to climax – they feel a forceful, and often inevitable, need to ejaculate. This is often known as the "point of no return". The rhythmic contractions at the base of the penis propel sperm and seminal fluid (combined to make semen) up the urethral tube and out of the penis tip.

During orgasm

The sperm are produced in the testicles and stored in the epididymis. Ejaculation begins with a series of contractions in the seminal vesicle, prostate gland, and rectum.

The sperm travels up via the vas deferens to the seminal vesicle. At the point of ejaculation, the contractions pump the sperm and seminal fluid (produced in the prostate gland) into the urethra, where they combine to make semen. Contractions in the penis force semen along to the urethral opening, where it is ejaculated.

After orgasm

Once orgasm occurs, a man goes into a refractory period where all the physical signs of sexual arousal drain from the body and he returns to his former relaxed,

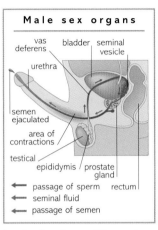

Male sex organs

vas deferens — bladder — seminal vesicle — urethra — semen ejaculated — area of contractions — testical — epididymis — prostate gland — rectum

← passage of sperm
← seminal fluid
← passage of semen

unstimulated state. The penis becomes limp. His heart rate, blood pressure, and sex flush subside, his breathing returns to normal, and the muscle tension is resolved. Unlike women, few men can repeat sexual intercourse immediately after orgasm, although multiple orgasms are possible in some men.

Her sexual response

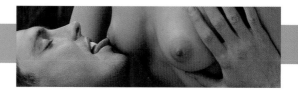

As with men, desire is the first stage of the female response cycle. A **sexy thought** enters a woman's brain, often triggered by touch, and the brain then transmits signals to **her genitals**. For women, **touch** and **desire** tend to be interrelated, and women are less likely to be turned on by a visual stimulus than men. Once **stimulation** begins and **excitement** builds, the woman starts to become **aroused** but this is a slower process than in men. Numerous changes start to take place in the body as it prepares for orgasm.

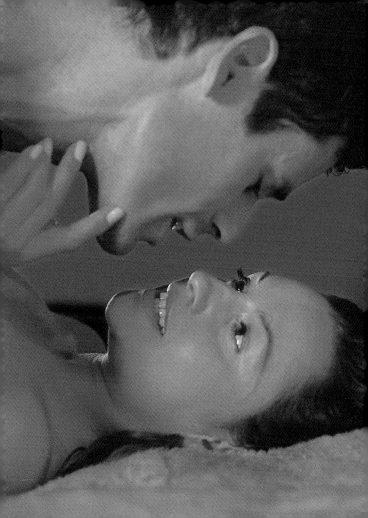

Becoming aroused

Arousal in women usually begins with the initial physical stimulation. Once a woman starts to get turned on (and just a passionate kiss can get the ball rolling), her breasts swell slightly and her nipples harden and, like her male partner, her muscles tense, her heart rate and blood pressure increase, and her breathing rate speeds up.

In preparation for intercourse, many changes occur in the genitals: the vagina becomes lubricated, in order to enable the penis to enter smoothly, then lengthens and swells with blood. This is similar to the male erection, although it is not as noticeable. In addition, the shape of the vagina alters slightly — this is known as "tenting", and occurs when the vaginal passage creates a kind of capped tent

shape. The labia also swell slightly as the sexual tension and excitement build. In fact, there is so much swelling of tissue around the clitoris that the clitoris seems to "disappear"

External signs

1 Prior to arousal, the clitoris, labia, and vagina are pink in colour and in a relaxed state. (After orgasm, it can take some time for the genitals to return to their normal shape and colour.)

2 When aroused, the vagina becomes lubricated, expands and swells with blood, and lengthens. The labia swell to three times their original thickness and move away from the vaginal opening.

3 When stimulated, the clitoris becomes enlarged and pulls back against the pubic bone. The clitoris may be difficult to see owing to the swelling of the surrounding tissues. The vagina and labia change in coloration from pink to a deep red or darker, purplish shade.

---

because it gets almost hidden. At this stage of extreme arousal, the tissues around the nipples swell with fluid so that nipple erection seems to disappear.

All-over body changes during arousal

When a woman is highly aroused, she may experience a sex flush that starts on the throat and abdomen and spreads to the breasts. Over one-third of women also perspire on the forehead, upper lip, chest, under the arms, and on the thighs and ankles. A thin layer of perspiration may also cover the back. As a woman becomes more aroused, involuntary muscular contractions also occur in the nipples (causing them to become erect), thighs, pelvis, back, abdomen, and feet.

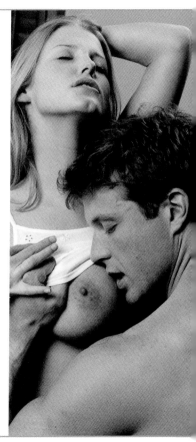

Reaching orgasm

Once tension and sensual feeling have built up sufficiently, orgasm is triggered. Contractions may be experienced in the vagina, clitoris, and uterus, as well as other body sites. Some women experience extra "wetness" during climax.

Most women, unlike men, are capable of holding off orgasm until they choose to experience one, and some can experience climax for a second or third time. A minority of women never experience orgasm, although this can sometimes be remedied by sex therapy.

After orgasm

Some women continue to remain sexually aroused after orgasm and can be stimulated again to experience further orgasms. Eventually though, the body relaxes and returns to its former resting state. The blood flow drains from the genitals, the heart rate and blood pressure subside, and breathing returns to normal. The sex flush lingers for a while but eventually disappears.

Female arousal

The time it takes for a woman to reach a state of extreme arousal can vary from a couple of minutes to three-quarters of an hour. During a high state of arousal, the vagina expands and tissue in the outer third of the vagina swells to form the orgasmic platform, which grips the penis during intercourse. The uterus rises and the clitoris retracts under its hood.

During orgasm, the cervix, uterus, and outer third of the vagina contract regularly. There are usually three to five (up to a maximum of 15) intensely pleasurable contractions at about 0.8 second intervals, although this varies.

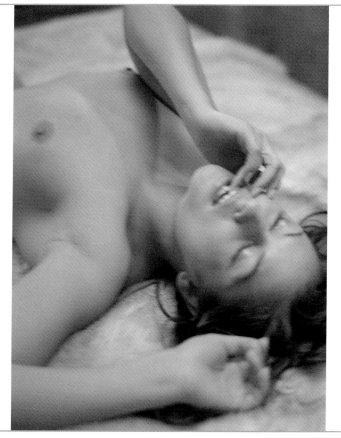

Orgasm techniques for him

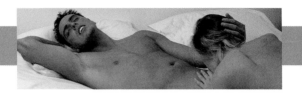

There's been so much written about **sex techniques for women** that men tend to get overlooked. Perhaps this is because they are lucky enough to become familiar with their genitals and **sexual response pattern** much earlier than most women. Nevertheless, male **experiences of orgasm** are just as individual as those of women and just as varied.

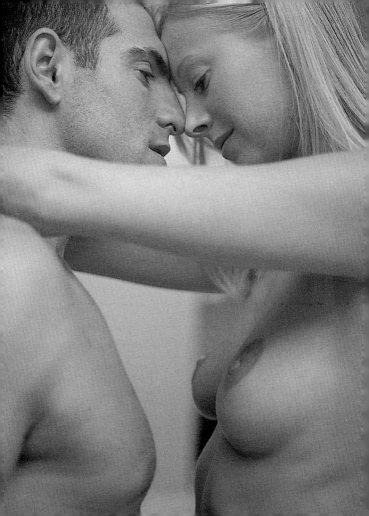

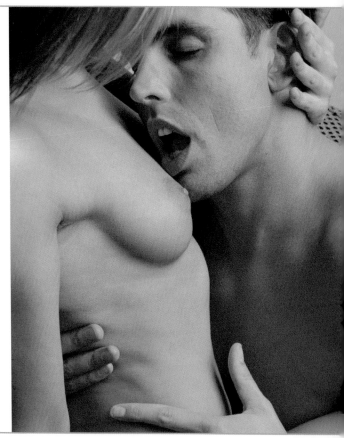

Orgasmic expectations

Although orgasm is virtually ensured for men in a way it is not for women, the sense of satisfaction from that same orgasm varies greatly. The man who yearns for a longer, stronger, and more intense experience may either have a lower sexual drive than most men or could be so anxious about his sexuality that he has physically exhausted himself with excessive sexual intercourse or masturbation. Alternatively, he may simply have unrealistic expectations of how amazing orgasm should be.

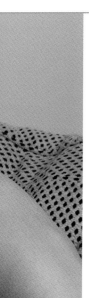

The way a man experiences orgasm differs between individuals. Some men are totally silent as they climax, while others call out or groan. As men age, the intensity of orgasm tends to diminish.

The pulsar

The pulsar is a technique that enhances the sensation of orgasm, and should be done during ejaculation. Clasp your two hands around the head of your man's penis. Squeeze gently, hold for a second then let go. Pause. Then do it again. The trick is to imitate the rhythm of the pulse. Try to time your pulsations to go with his contractions.

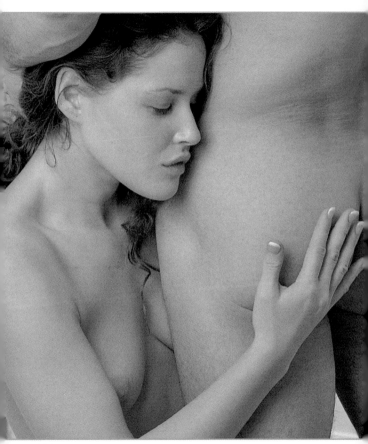

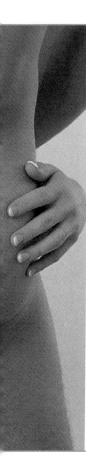

**Work up
to it slowly**
Try to take
stimulation slowly.
A man becomes
aroused more
quickly than a
woman, so if
his climax comes
too soon she will
miss out.

Stimulate the prostate

This tends to be the man's
forgotten sex organ, mainly
because it is hidden at the top of
the anal passage. Yet stimulation
of the prostate alone, through
massage, can bring a man to
orgasm. There are now some
excellent anal vibrators designed
for this task (see p.142).

Locating the prostate

The prostate gland
encircles the urethra at
the exit from the bladder.
To reach it, insert a well-
lubricated finger into the
anus and press against its
front wall (the side nearest
the penis). You will feel
the prostate gland as a
firm, walnut-sized mass.
Press it in a sustained,
regular rhythm to give
maximum pleasure.
Always wash your hands
immediately afterwards.

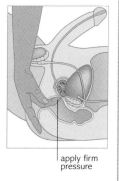

apply firm
pressure

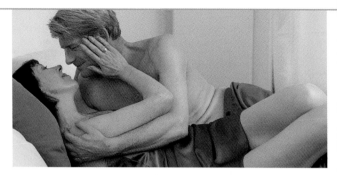

Age and experience

Most young men experience little difficulty with climax, except possibly that it happens too fast (see pp.208–209). Generally, the younger you are, the easier, stronger, and more copious in terms of ejaculation the orgasm will be. Men are believed to be at their sexual peak at around the age of 18. Ten years later, at the age of 28, that orgasmic experience will have already changed, and will continue to do so as the man ages. Although the orgasmic experience will still continue to feel intensely pleasurable, it will not be as long or as strong as in the early years. Nor will it be desired so often. For some men who identify closely with their sexual response, this can sometimes be distressing. However, we need to recognize that this is a perfectly natural part of the ageing process, and that by keeping healthy and fit we can extend our sexual life.

10 tips to improve orgasm

Orgasms provide fantastic sensations. Here are a few tips that will make them even better:

1 Delay climax – the more drawn out the build-up to sex, the more sexual tension there is to release at the time of orgasm, leading to a deeper climax. There are a number of delaying techniques you can try (see pp.232–233).

2 Do exercises to develop muscle control so that you can time your climaxes better. These will also increase your chances of experiencing multiple orgasms (see p.96).

3 Include the prostate gland in your stimulation, either before or during intercourse (see left).

4 Stroke and caress the perineum and testicles sensitively – they are highly erogenous zones.

5 Use your imagination: think sexy thoughts, remember sexy sights, and go to places in your mind where you wouldn't dream of going in real life.

6 Abstain from alcohol, tobacco, and drugs. These can all dull sexual sensation and adversely affect performance.

7 Improve penile muscle tone through exercises such as pelvic-floor exercises (see p.223)

8 Use first-class sex lubrication. A lubricated penis instantly becomes more sensitive and receives more pleasurable feeling than a dry one.

9 Experiment with the pulsar technique (see p.207), which feels fantastic during ejaculation.

10 Try climaxing in only one out of three lovemaking sessions – the belief is that in this way you can build up an explosive orgasm and intense sensation.

Orgasm techniques for her

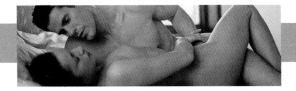

Most informed young men today know that the movement of penile thrusting alone may well not bring their loved one to the **heights of ecstasy**. So what are the main methods of her **enjoyng orgasm**? A woman's climax depends primarily on the amount of **stimulation** her **clitoris** receives – her clitoris being the main **organ** of **sensation**.

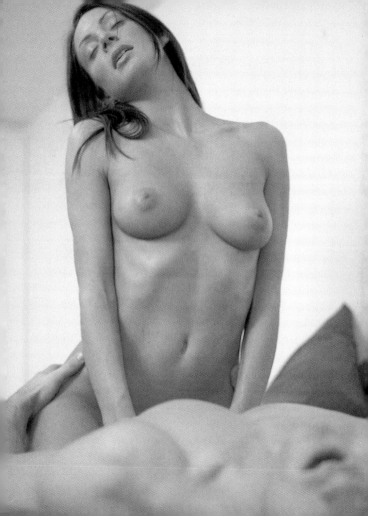

Intercourse plus masturbation

Intercourse alone isn't usually the best way for a woman to enjoy an orgasm. This is because the clitoris doesn't get enough direct stimulation from the penis. It appears to be a design fault in the human female that the clitoris is situated so high on the genitals it tends to get missed by the thrust of lovemaking.

Of the women who do manage to climax during intercourse, we now know that the in–out movement of the penis exerts a mild downward pull of the clitoral hood, which is attached to the labia, on the sensitive clitoris. For some women this slight stimulation is enough. But for most, it is not. Indeed, some women never experience orgasm from intercourse alone.

The majority of women want and enjoy intercourse but need that something extra to make it finally culminate in a climax. The most straightforward way is to give your lover a lot of stimulation by hand so that she is extremely aroused by the time you get to intercourse. For some women, this is enough to get them up and over into orgasm. Others need the manual stimulation continued even during intercourse. This stimulation can be done either by him or by her and is extremely effective.

During the first six months of a new sexual relationship, a couple are likely to experiment with many different sex positions, partly to discover what feels best for this particular

Guiding him
Every woman's sexual response is different, so it's important that the woman guides her partner and communicates how and where she likes to be touched.

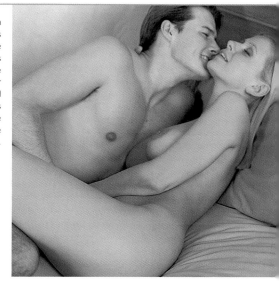

couple combination. Experimenting with sex from the rear, for example, is one sex position couples regularly try out, but it can sometimes prove very disappointing for the woman because she doesn't have an orgasm this way. The reason for this is that her clitoris gets no stimulation at all from this position. However, there is an easy answer to this – the man can reach his fingers around and masturbate her at the same time. It can feel exciting, erotic, and very arousing.

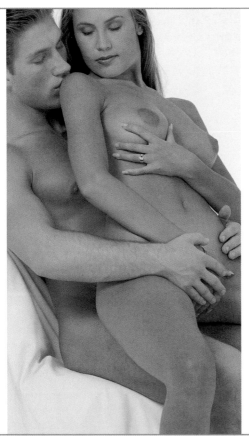

Extra stimulation
Some women require manual stimulation in order to continue to climax during intercourse. Here, the man reaches his hand around and stimulates her clitoris, timing the touch to his thrusts.

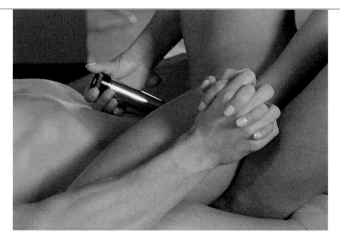

The joy of vibrators

There are some men and women for whom the combination of masturbation and intercourse either feels uncomfortable or still does not offer enough stimulation. This is where vibrators come to the rescue (see pp.138–139). Vibrators are not just for novelty value; for some women they are essential, and can make the difference between experiencing orgasm and never doing so. Vibrators today have travelled a long way from the pink plastic, penis-shaped models. You can purchase them in bright jelly colours, in a variety of shapes and sizes, and with a number of special and very pleasing attributes.

The G-spot

The G-spot is a small area on the front wall of the vagina, although it doesn't appear to be present in all women. When pressed, it is believed to trigger orgasm. It is named after gynaecologist Ernst Grafenburg, who first described it, relating it to the point where the urethra runs closest to the top of the vaginal wall. Others think it to be the vestiges of what would have been the prostate gland if the foetus had developed into a

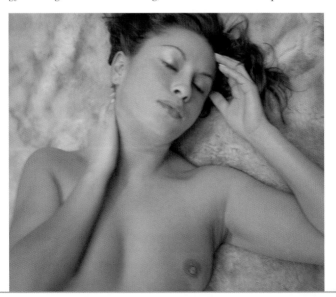

boy. Indeed, some women who appear to have G-spot orgasm appear to ejaculate a thin arc of fluid, which has proved to be similar to seminal fluid, when climaxing. The latest theory is that the G-spot is the root of the clitoris – hence its sensitivity.

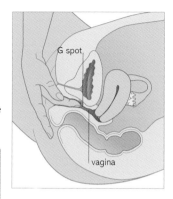

Sex for one

Most women love the closeness and fullness they experience during face-to-face intercourse. However, they may not necessarily get intense climaxes this way. Self-touch generally offers much longer, stronger, more drawn-out orgasmic experiences. It's a good idea to experience self-stimulation so that you learn your own orgasmic patterns as well as your own erogenous zones. If you know what gives you an orgasm, you can take this information into your relationship and help your man find his way.

How to stimulate the G-spot

Exert a steady pressure with your finger on the spot, pushing for a count of ten, then let go, then press again. It is pressure rather than light stroking that brings on the erotic sensation and can trigger climax.

Place your finger inside your vagina and try to reach the far end (this can be very difficult). Reach with the finger towards your abdomen. The G-spot feels like a small bump swelling out of the front wall of the vagina.

Multiple orgasms

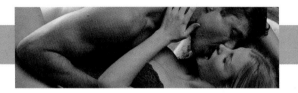

Women have long been known to be capable of **multiple orgasms**. In the 1940s, the **Kinsey Report** revealed that 14 per cent of women interviewed experienced multiple climaxes, and Masters and Johnson's scientific laboratory research in the 1950s confirmed that this was **certainly possible**. It is now believed that some **men** may be **capable** of **more than one orgasm** in a session.

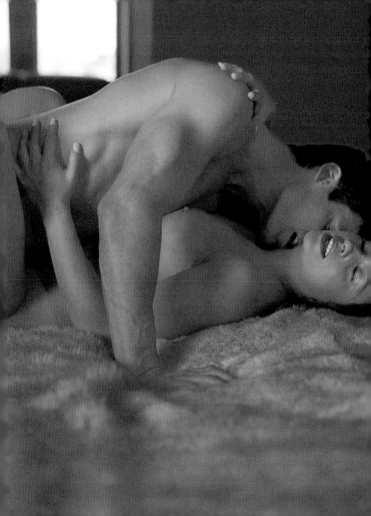

Multiple orgasms for men

Laboratory research carried out by American sex researchers Hartman and Fithian in the 1970s indicated that men may be capable of experiencing multiple orgasms, and that their orgasms may or may not involve ejaculation. Since male climax is so associated with ejaculation, no one can say for certain whether the multi-orgasmic males observed were actually climaxing or if they were simply experiencing peaks of excitement. Whatever the case, they were clearly undergoing an extremely intense, prolonged sexual experience – their breathing quickened, their heart rate increased, and their muscle tension intensified. One of the subjects appeared to have seven distinct orgasms in ten minutes.

The men managed their multiple climaxes by self-control and training: they tensed their thighs and squeezed their pelvic-floor muscles, thus blocking off their ejaculations by closing their urethral tubes with muscle action.

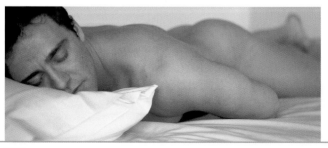

Multiple orgasm training for men

There are various ways you can develop the right degree of muscle control to achieve multiple orgasms, although it does take time and patience:

1 Learn testicle control. Standing with your feet apart, pull up your testicle muscles towards your lower abdomen. Repeat as often as possible every day, but stop if your testicles begin to hurt.

2 Give yourself an erection and train yourself to keep it hard for as long as possible.

3 Climax is triggered by a kind of tension in the pelvic area called "myotonia". To build this up, alternately flex and relax your thighs and lower abdomen for as long as possible: five minutes is the aim, but stop if you get cramp.

4 Excite yourself slowly, building up to a high pitch of arousal over a long time. When you feel about to reach orgasm, clench your pelvic-floor muscles. If you feel this isn't going to work, try the Beautrais manoeuvre (see p.232), in which you pull down on your testicles, or the squeeze technique (see p.233), which involves squeezing the penis.

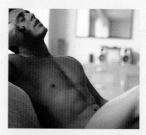

Multiple orgasm exercises
To build up muscle tension in the pelvic area, alternately flex and relax your lower abdomen, pelvic-floor muscles, and thighs.

Multiple orgasms for women

Not all women experience multiple orgasms, but a lot more can manage it than their male counterparts. Multiple climaxes can be experienced in various ways, but they tend to consist of a series of separate orgasms occurring within a short time, sometimes with only a few seconds between, occasionally longer. Some women experience them as a series of gentle peaks of excitement that feel connected, while others have one strong climax after another.

No one yet knows why some women should be able to have multiple climaxes and not others, although carrying on with stimulation is essential. One theory is that the more testosterone you have, the more likely you are to climax easily and often.

Taking medication

Certain medications, such as the contraceptive pill, can lessen sexual response. If you have taken the Pill all your sexual life, it might be more difficult to determine if you can have multiple climaxes.

Sex tip

Don't see it as a personal failure if you don't achieve multiple orgasms. Nearly all men and many women never experience them, and this is perfectly normal.

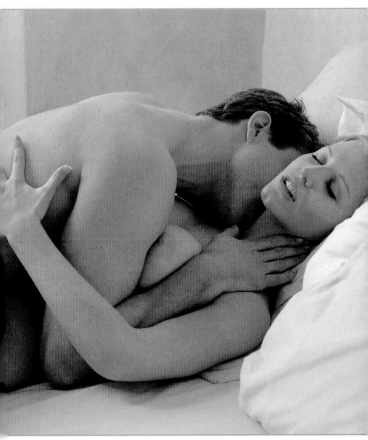

How to have multiple orgasms

To experience multiple orgasms a woman must always have continued stimulation after her initial climax – it is vital to maintain a high degree of arousal. Her partner needs either to continue intercourse, or to press on with manual stimulation, instead of stopping because he thinks

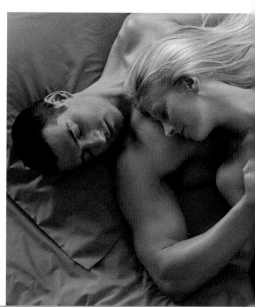

Maintaining excitement
After your first orgasm, keep up the stimulation. At the very least you may discover that your orgasm can continue for far longer than you anticipated. At best, it may turn into more than one.

her climax is over. If you are experimenting on yourself, instead of removing your fingers from your clitoris because it feels so sensitive after orgasm, carry on with the stimulation. You could also use a vibrator to experiment with prolonging stimulation after the first climax.

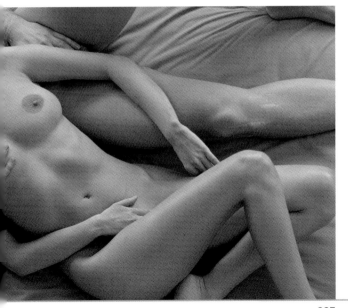

Controlling orgasms

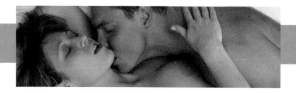

Timing tends to be a crucial element of good sex, because it is frequently the key to whether or not both partners experience **orgasm**. With the right element of control, a couple can prolong the **sexual experience** and can vary the type of orgasm they wish to experience, for example a **simultaneous orgasm**, when both partners climax at the same time; a sequential one, when one partner's orgasm follows the other; or even **multiple orgasms**, where the woman (and occasionally man) have several climaxes in quick succession.

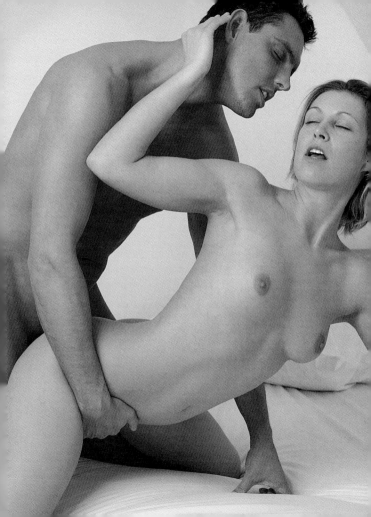

Types of orgasms

Prior to all the ground-breaking sexual research of the 1960s and 1970s, the belief was that the "correct" way to experience orgasm was at the same time as your partner. Indeed, having an orgasm at the same moment as your lover can feel extremely intimate. However, many people prefer a sequential orgasm to a simultaneous one since this allows you to enjoy the intensity of your own experience rather than being distracted by thinking of your partner's enjoyment at such a crucial point.

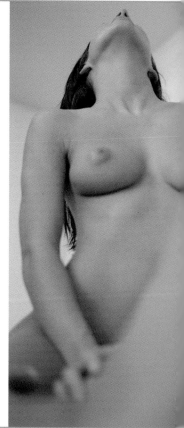

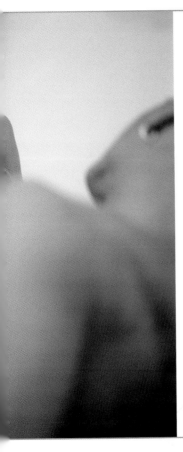

Since most men cannot continue intercourse after ejaculation, and because most women tend to need more stimulation than their man, the best way to experience simultaneous orgasm is to excite your woman first until she reaches a point of arousal that appears to match your own. Let go of your own climax only when she is clearly almost at the point of climax too.

Sex tip

Women – to encourage orgasm or to enhance the experience, try thinking of scenes from a sexy story or fantasy, or an erotic film.

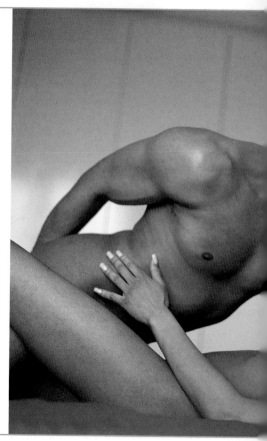

Beautrais manoeuvre
To prolong intercourse, when you feel that you're on the brink of orgasm, grasp your testicles and pull down very firmly. This has the effect of blocking the urethral passage and so prevents ejaculation.

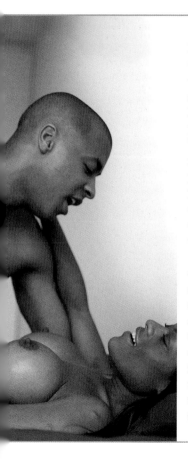

Delaying male orgasm

In order to ensure that your woman reaches orgasm, or that the two of you climax simultaneously, you need to have complete control of your penis to get the timing right. This can be difficult for many men specially those who prematurely ejaculate. It is particularly important for these men to slow themselves down, or their partners may never get the chance to reach orgasm.

Fortunately, orgasm control can be learned. You could try and improve your muscle control by doing exercises. Alternatively, control climax using the Beautrais manoeuvre, or the squeeze technique, which involves squeezing the ridge on the penis head firmly between the thumb and forefingers at the point of no return.

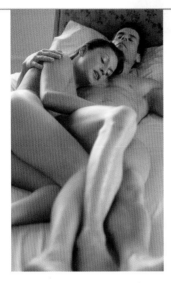

Delaying orgasm for women

One of the sex differences between men and women is that if you stop stimulating a man, he remains sexually excited. If you stop stimulating a woman, her arousal fades so rapidly that it takes quite a while to bring her back to the same peak of excitement.

So if you are one of those rare women who climaxes too soon, try stopping the stimulation for a short time and giving your man oral sex or manual stimulation for a while. It should slow you down without materially affecting your partner.

Sex tip

Tantric sex (see pp.76–83) aims at slowing down and intensifying the orgasmic experience, and side-by-side positions (see pp.40–45) can also be slow and sensual and so likely to prolong intercourse and delay orgasm.

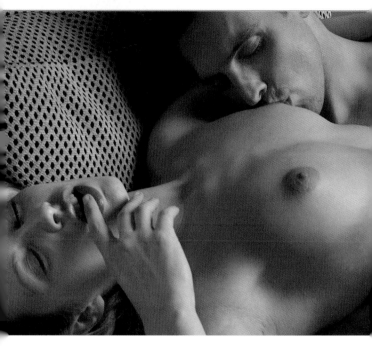

Bring her to climax

To give your woman maximum pleasure, concentrate on stimulating her and hold back your own orgasm. When she is ready, either bring her to orgasm first, or time it so that you climax together.

Index

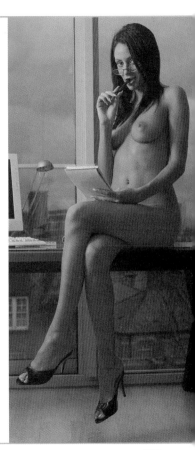

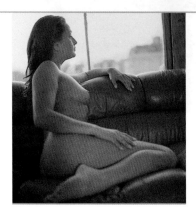

Acknowledgments

The publisher would like to thank
Sh! Women's Erotic Emporium and
Master U for the supply of materials,
Contance Novice for proofreading,
and Hilary Bird for the index.

Photography: Luc Beziat,
James Muldowney, Peter Pugh-Cook
Illustrations: Richard Tibbits, John Geary
All images © Dorling Kindersley
For further information see:
www.dkimages.com